NCLEX Takeover

Achieve Mastery in Lab Values, Fluids, and
Electrolytes (4 Book Boxset)

Chase Hassen

Nurse Superhero

© 2015

Disclaimer:

Although the author and publisher have made every effort to ensure that the information in this book was correct at press time, the author and publisher do not assume and hereby disclaim any liability to any party for any loss, damage, or disruption caused by errors or omissions, whether such errors or omissions result from negligence, accident, or any other cause.

This book is not intended as a substitute for the medical advice of physicians. The reader should regularly consult a physician in matters relating to his/her health and particularly with respect to any symptoms that may require diagnosis or medical attention.

Table of Contents

Get my book FREE now!

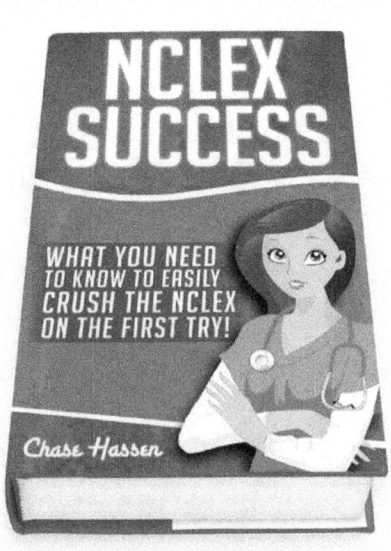

Just to say thanks for downloading my book, I wanted to give you another resource to help you absolutely crush the NCLEX Exam.

For a limited time you can download this book for FREE.

http://bit.ly/1VNGAZ9

Lab Values

137 Values You Must Know to Easily Pass the NCLEX!

Chase Hassen

Nurse Superhero

© 2015

Table of Contents

Chapter 1: Introduction to Lab Values

Nearly all hospitalized patients, many emergency department patients, and some outpatient patients will have one or more lab values taken as part of their care. Labs are generally taken from a peripheral vein or from urine samples. A few labs, by necessity, must be taken from a peripheral artery in order to get accurate measurements of arterial oxygen and acid-base measurements. In infants, blood is often drawn from a very vascular heel stick. Things like blood glucose and Hemoglobin A1C can be done on a finger stick.

Most of the time, the labs come back through medical records and are initially read by the nursing staff. This means that you, the nurse, are often the first person to make a medical determination of what the lab values mean. This is why it is important to know as much as you can about lab values so that pertinent ones can be passed onto the healthcare provider/doctor as soon as possible.

Lab values vary according to the machine being used by a particular lab facility so, when in doubt, refer to the reference values listed along with the labs. The laboratory reference ranges given in this book will be as close as possible to the accepted reference ranges but might differ slightly from the reference ranges you receive along with the laboratory values.

Labs tell a lot about what is going on with the patient from the inside of their body and often are more enlightening than the vital signs and physical examination. This is why laboratory values are among the most important things to obtain from a sick patient. Labs tell the biochemistry of what is going on in the body and their interpretation is crucial to many diagnoses given to the patient.

How are Lab Values Obtained?

In larger facilities, lab draws are done by laboratory professionals but it is still an important thing for nurses to know how to do.

Blood is usually taken from a peripheral vein, usually in the antecubital fossa or on the back of the hands. When doing this procedure, it is a good idea to apply a rubber tourniquet proximal to the blood draw site, telling the patient that it will feel tight while the blood is being drawn. Wipe down potential veins with an alcohol swab. Swabbing vigorously will sometimes enlarge the vein and make it easier to obtain the specimen. With the bevel side up, insert the needle into the vein. You can use a vacutainer needle, which has a barrel for inserting vacuum-created vials, or a butterfly needle for small and more delicate veins. For really difficult-to-get veins, you can attach the butterfly needle to a large syringe so that you can gradually "milk" the blood from the vein.

When you have enough blood, apply a cotton ball to the site and remove the needle, asking the patient to hold pressure on the site (if possible), while you label the vials and put the needle in a biohazard container. You need to check to make sure the bleeding has stopped and tape the cotton ball tightly to the vein site. Those people who are on anticoagulants such as warfarin, heparin, and aspirin may require prolonged direct pressure of up to 10 minutes after drawing blood.

For a heel stick in a baby, several drops of blood can be taken. You start by cleansing the heel with an alcohol swab. Using a sterile lancet, pierce the heel and squeeze the heel gently to allow for the expression of how many droplets of blood you need to get out. The blood can be placed into a small vial or onto blotter paper (as is done for neonatal testing). Apply pressure to the puncture site until the bleeding stops and then apply a Band-Aid. Tell the patient's parents to leave the bandage on for at least a half hour and make sure they know that there might be bruising at the site of the puncture wound.

For a finger stick, pick a finger and cleanse the distal phalangeal area with an alcohol swab. Pierce the finger on the side or pad of the finger with a lancet. Collect as much as is recommended into a small test tube, milking the finger drop-by-drop. If a blood sugar is being obtained, wipe off the first drop with a piece of gauze or a cotton ball and allow the glucose meter to "suck up" the drop of blood into the test strip. Put pressure for 30 seconds to a minute at the site of the puncture wound. You may need to apply a Band-Aid if the bleeding does not stop spontaneously.

For an arterial blood stick, the blood is usually taken from the radial artery in the wrist. This is a relatively difficult procedure to accomplish so you might have to defer this task to the physician or laboratory attendant. The radial artery is palpated by checking the pulse in the wrist. With the palm side up, alcohol is used to cover the area to be punctured. The needle and syringe are inserted at a

90 degree angle to the skin until the needle reaches the artery. Inform the patient that this is a relatively painful procedure but that it won't take long and they must remain still so the procedure can go as planned. When the needle reaches the artery, the syringe will fill by itself. Put the syringe and needle combination on ice for the trip to the laboratory. You need to apply pressure to the puncture site for up to ten minutes.

Remember that drawing blood involves the possibility of contact with biohazardous substances. Wear gloves while drawing blood and throw all needles and sharps into a designated biohazard container. When the container is full, have it exchanged for an empty one; do not keep stuffing things into an already-filled biohazard container. If you get a finger poke or other poke from a contaminated needle, tell your supervisor and follow your organizations regulations for becoming in contact with a potential biohazard.

Chapter 2: The Basic Chemistry Panel

The definition of "basic chemistry panel" varies from institution to institution. You can just order electrolytes as part of a basic chemistry panel, while some labs offer BUN, creatinine and other labs as part of the panel. Others add serum protein levels along with electrolytes.

Almost all chemistry panels include a set of electrolytes, namely the sodium, potassium, and chloride. These labs are important to understanding the fluid and electrolyte balance in the body. Other electrolytes often used as part of a chemistry panel are magnesium, calcium, and phosphorus.

Electrolytes are metal salts that are either positively or negatively charged, depending on their chemical characteristics. Electrolytes are pumped inside and outside the cells and the body attempts to maintain homeostasis as much as possible. Blood is taken from the patient's vein and spun to spin out the cells so that only plasma remains. The serum of the blood is defined as the plasma minus the clotting factors. Tests on the electrolytes as part of a basic chemistry panel are done on serum.

Calcium

Calcium is mainly stored in the bones and teeth with a lesser amount flowing in the bloodstream. Calcium and phosphorus levels are closely linked in that, as the calcium level increases, the phosphorus level drops. This is due to the action of the parathyroid hormone (PTH), secreted by the parathyroid glands imbedded in thyroid tissue in the neck. As PTH levels rise, so does the serum chloride level. PTH also causes an uptake of vitamin D that increases calcium absorption from the diet. You need vitamin D in order to absorb calcium from the GI tract. If, on the other hand, the calcium level is too high, calcitonin is released by the thyroid gland, causing the calcium levels to drop. Calcium can be measured as the total calcium level, including that which is bound to albumin and "ionized calcium" levels, which is the unbound calcium.

Calcium levels are checked whenever there is concern for parathyroid gland dysfunction or overactivity, kidney function, kidney stones, bone diseases, certain cancers and pancreatitis. Low calcium blood levels can cause depression, muscle spasms, tingling around the mouth, confusion and muscle twitching. High calcium levels cause bony pain, nausea, vomiting, weakness poor appetite, abdominal pain, constipation and increased urine output.

The normal non-ionized calcium level is approximately 9.0 to 10.5 mg/dL in adults. Children have a slightly different reference range at 7.6 to 10.8 mg/dL. Ionized calcium levels are about 4.65-5.28 mg/dL.

High calcium levels may indicate tuberculosis, prolonged bed rest, kidney disease, elevated PTH, cancer metastasized to bone, Addison's disease, dehydration, elevated thyroid hormone, Paget's disease, sarcoidosis, liver disease, decreased phosphate, and ingesting too much calcium. Low calcium levels indicate low PTH levels, high phosphorus levels, low albumin levels, malabsorption syndrome, pancreatitis, low magnesium, or kidney disease.

Magnesium

Magnesium is generally stored in cells and in bone. It helps the transfer of potassium and sodium into and out of the cells. Fluctuation of magnesium causes muscle weakness, twitching of muscles, arrhythmias, nausea, vomiting, dizziness and low blood pressure. Normal magnesium levels are about 1.3-2.1 mEq/L. In children, the normal levels are 1.4-1.7 mEq/L.

Elevated levels of magnesium occur in hyperparathyroidism, hypothyroidism, Addison's disease, kidney failure, dehydration, taking too much antacid medication and laxatives containing magnesium. Low levels of magnesium can be seen in pancreatitis, diabetic ketoacidosis, hypercalcemia, alcohol abuse, alcohol withdrawal, celiac sprue, starvation, low intake of magnesium, elevated calcium levels, kidney disease, hyperthyroidism, burns, preeclampsia, and starvation.

Phosphorus

Phosphorus is found in the body as the phosphate ion. It is used for growing bones and teeth and is a part of muscle contraction. Phosphate levels rise as calcium levels drop. Phosphate is used to screen for kidney disease, bone disease and for functioning of the parathyroid gland. The normal range for phosphate is 3.0-4.5 mg/dL in adults or 4.5-6.5 mg/dL in children.

Elevated phosphate levels are seen in acromegaly, pregnancy, low PTH, low vitamin D, osteomalacia, malnutrition, liver disease, low vitamin D levels, celiac sprue, elevated calcium levels, and burns. Low levels of phosphate are seen in elevated calcium situations, high PTH, poor nutrition, low vitamin D levels, and alcohol abuse.

Potassium

Potassium is normally stored inside the cells so there is much less in the bloodstream. It is responsible for muscle contraction, fluid balance, and nerve transmission. Its concentration is regulated by the release of aldosterone, secreted by the adrenal glands. As the potassium level goes up, the sodium level goes down and vice versa. The normal level of potassium in adults is 3.5-5.0 mEq/L. The level in children is 3.4-4.7 mEq/L. High levels are found in excess intake of potassium, myocardial infarction, the taking of ACE inhibitors, kidney disease or diabetic ketoacidosis. Low levels are seen when taking certain diuretics, increased aldosterone levels, diarrhea, alcoholism, cystic fibrosis, vomiting, malnutrition, dehydration, and burns.

Sodium

Sodium is also regulated by aldosterone secreted by the adrenal glands. There is a higher concentration of sodium in the bloodstream than is found in the cells with an inverse relationship between sodium and potassium. It is tested whenever a there is a need for electrolyte balance assessment and for the presence of adrenal disease. The normal range is between 136 and 145 mEq/L. High levels of sodium as seen in Cushing's syndrome, diabetic ketoacidosis, kidney dysfunction, dehydration, elevated sodium intake, diabetes insipidus, diarrhea, vomiting, and elevated aldosterone levels. Low sodium levels are found in psychogenic polydipsia, vomiting, diarrhea, burns, heart failure, malnutrition, liver cirrhosis, kidney disease, and low aldosterone levels.

Chloride

Chloride is found mainly outside of the cells and mimics the sodium level. Abnormalities of chloride are seen in metabolic acidosis, adrenal gland problems, and kidney disease. The normal levels of chloride are 98-106 mEq/L in adults and 90-110 mEq/L in children. High levels of chloride are seen in anemia, kidney disease, dehydration, increased PTH, and salt ingestion. Low levels are seen in burns, kidney failure, heart failure, Cushing's syndrome, vomiting, syndrome of inappropriate ADH secretion and diabetic ketoacidosis.

Serum Proteins

A measure of the total serum protein level assesses the amount of albumin, globulin and other proteins in the bloodstream. A comparison of albumin to globulin is also made. The main protein found in the bloodstream is albumin, while globulin is produced as part of the immune system. Albumin is made by the liver; it keeps blood from leaking out of the blood vessels and is a carrier for other molecules in the bloodstream. Globulin comes in three forms: alpha, beta, and gamma. Protein levels are part of a screening test for liver/kidney dysfunction, malnutrition, as well as the cause of ascites, edema and pulmonary edema. The normal total protein level is 6.0-8.3 g/dL. High protein levels are seen in chronic infections or chronic inflammations, Waldenstrom's disease, and multiple myeloma. Low total protein levels are seen in bleeding, extensive burns, agammaglobulinemia, glomerulonephritis, malabsorption, malnutrition, liver disease, protein-losing enteropathies and nephrotic syndrome.

Chapter 3: Liver and Kidney Function

The liver and kidneys are the major organs in the system when it comes to the myriad of processes that regulate protein levels, electrolyte levels, and waste products in the body. This is why many chemistry profiles include the basic function of both the liver and the kidneys.

Kidney Function Studies

Kidney function studies include the BUN, creatinine, urine creatinine and creatinine clearance. Each is a valuable test of kidney function and can tell whether or not the kidneys are doing their job.

BUN (Blood urea nitrogen)

This measures the amount of urea nitrogen, which is the product of protein breakdown. The normal BUN level is 6-20 mg/dL. Abnormal BUN levels will show up with the following conditions:
1. High protein levels in the GI tract

2. Congestive heart failure

3. GI bleeding

4. Dehydration

5. Kidney disease

6. Urinary tract blockage

7. Heart attack

8. Shock

Low levels of BUN will show up in these conditions:
2. Low protein in the diet

3. Liver failure

4. Over-hydration

5. Malnutrition

Creatinine (Blood)

Creatinine levels reflect the overall functioning of the kidneys. Certain medications can interfere with the creatinine level including cimetidine, aminoglycosides, chemotherapy using heavy metals, trimethoprim, and NSAID therapy. Creatinine is a waste product of the molecule creatine in the body. Creatine supplies energy to muscles and other tissue. Creatinine is exclusively removed by the kidneys and if kidney failure is present, the creatinine level will rise. A normal level for creatinine is 0.7-1.3 mg/dL in men and 0.6-1.1 mg/dL in females.

Elevated serum creatinine levels are associated with kidney failure or kidney damage, a blocked urinary tract, dehydration, rhabdomyolysis, preeclampsia or eclampsia (in pregnancy). People with myasthenia gravis and end stage muscular dystrophy will also have an elevated creatinine.

Creatinine Clearance

This is a test of the function of the kidneys. It is a test that makes a comparison between the creatinine in the blood and the creatinine in the urine. As part of the test, the urinary and blood creatinine levels are taken. The urine is collected over a twenty-four hour period of time. The test measures the glomerular filtration rate or GFR. This is a measure of how well the kidneys filter the blood. The creatinine clearance in normal people is 97-137 ml/min in males and 88-128 ml/min in females.

An abnormal creatinine clearance level can tell whether or not there is damage to the filtering tubular cells of the kidney in kidney diseases and kidney failure. It can also be low if there is diminished blood flow to the kidneys, dehydration, heart failure and outflow obstruction in the bladder.

Urine Creatinine Level

This is a measure of the amount of creatinine found in the urine. In order to do the test, the urine must be collected in a jug for twenty-four hours. Certain medications can interfere with the test, including some antibiotic, cisplatin, and cimetidine. It is a test that can help tell whether or not the kidneys are filtering properly. It is performed as a part of the creatinine clearance test. The urine creatinine level ranges from 500-2000 mg per day, depending on how old you are and on the amount of lean body mass you have.

Elevated amounts of creatinine in the urine can be found in high meat diets, kidney damage, lack of blood flow to the kidneys, kidney failure, rhabdomyolysis, and obstruction of the urinary tract.

Glomerular Filtration Rate

The GFR or glomerular filtration rate is a test of kidney function. The test estimates how much blood is passing through the glomeruli every minute. It is a blood test that uses the creatinine level to estimate the GFR by using a formula based on age, creatinine, ethnicity, weight, height, and gender.

The test is often done to assess kidney failure in those who have a family history of kidney disease, diabetes, heart disease, bladder infections, hypertension and urinary blockage. A normal GFR is between 90 and 110 ml/min. GFR decreases with age. GFR levels less than 60 ml/min indicate the presence of some degree of chronic renal failure. The lower the GFR, the greater is the degree of chronic renal failure.

Liver Function Tests

The liver is responsible for many different things including the production of bile salts and the metabolism of proteins and toxic waste products. It stores glucose in the form of glycogen. Liver failure is extremely dangerous but there are tests that can be done to assess the degree of liver cell damage and cellular function. As the largest gland in the body, the liver is also responsible for making albumin for the body and making clotting factors. The liver metabolizes red blood cell proteins into bilirubin, which is then cleared from the body through the urine or stool.

Alanine Aminotransferase (ALT)

This test used to be called the SGPT test. It is an enzyme found in the liver, heart, muscles, kidneys and pancreas. Liver damage causes ALT to be released into the bloodstream, increasing the level. ALT and another test, the AST together can detect the presence of liver disease. These two tests are done along with the LDH test and bilirubin level to assess the functioning of the liver. Certain things, like strenuous exercise, the taking of some herbal remedies and pregnancy can affect the ALT level. Because ALT is produced by other body organs, it must be interpreted in light of the other test results and the clinical findings. A normal ALT level is between 4 and 36 U/L. Mildly high levels can be seen in cirrhosis, fatty liver, and the taking of certain medications, including statin drugs, antibiotics, barbiturates, chemotherapy and narcotics. Moderately elevated levels are seen in acetaminophen abuse and alcohol abuse. High levels are seen in mononucleosis, necrosis of the liver, hepatitis, lead poisoning, shock, and rapid progression of acute lymphocytic leukemia in a child.

Alkaline Phosphatase (ALP)

ALP is an enzyme produced by the liver, bones, intestines, kidneys and the placenta. It is interpreted along with other liver tests to determine whether or not the elevation in ALP is associated with liver damage. Birth control pills, antibiotics, certain diabetic medications and aspirin can adversely affect the ALP levels. In a child and in post-menopausal women, the ALP can be elevated with a normal liver. The normal ALP level is between 30 and 126 U/L. In children, the ALT level can be as high as 300 U/L. Very high levels can be seen in obstructive jaundice, gallbladder disease, hepatitis, liver disease, rickets, osteomalacia, Paget disease of bone, and metastatic cancer to bone. It is also elevated in infectious mononucleosis, hyperparathyroidism, renal cancer heart failure and a heart attack. Low levels can be seen in malnutrition, celiac disease, and scurvy. High levels can also normally be seen in the third trimester of pregnancy because of placental secretion of ALP. Children experiencing a rapid growth rate will have an elevated ALT level because of bone growth.

Ammonia

Ammonia is made by intestinal bacteria as they break down proteins. Ammonia is then further broken down in the liver to make urea, eventually excreted in the urine. If the ammonia level is elevated, it means the liver cannot convert the ammonia to urea. Patients with severe cirrhosis of the liver or liver failure will have elevated ammonia levels. Symptoms of elevated ammonia level include sleepiness, confusion, coma or hand tremors. Many medications can contribute to elevated ammonia levels. A normal ammonia level is between 15 and 45 mcg/dL in adults and 40-80 mcg/dL in children. Common causes of an elevated ammonia level include hepatitis, cirrhosis of the liver, intestinal or stomach bleeding, heart failure, kidney failure and in hemolytic disease of the newborn.

Aspartate aminotransferase (AST)

This used to be called the SGOT test and is an enzyme found in the heart, liver, kidneys, red blood cells, muscle tissue and pancreas. The test must therefore be interpreted in light of the other liver tests and clinical findings. It is a more effective test for the determination of liver failure and liver damage than is the ALT. Like the AST test, it can be thrown off by strenuous exercise or the taking of some herbal supplements. High vitamin A doses can affect the AST. A normal range of AST is 8-35 U/L. There can be slightly elevated levels in fatty liver disease, alcohol abuse, acetaminophen abuse, chemotherapy, barbiturate use or narcotic use. Kidney damage, muscular dystrophy, lung damage, elevated vitamin A intake, heart failure, heart attack, myositis, mononucleosis, and certain cancers can elevate the AST. High levels of AST are seen in shock, viral hepatitis, burns, drug reactions, liver trauma, pulmonary embolism, heatstroke, poisoning, and liver necrosis.

Bilirubin

Bilirubin is the waste product of the breakdown of red blood cells. It forms the brown color of bile and is what gives stool the brownish color. There is indirect (unconjugated) bilirubin and direct (conjugated) bilirubin. The liver turns unconjugated bilirubin into water soluble direct bilirubin. The blood test for bilirubin measures both the total and direct bilirubin levels. Indirect bilirubin is calculated from the other two values. The bilirubin test is a good measure of liver and gallbladder function. Neonatal jaundice is usually caused by a slow transfer of indirect to direct bilirubin in the newborn period that turns around when the liver kicks in. Medications like Valium, Dilantin, birth control pills, indomethacin, or Dalmane can raise bilirubin levels. Other medications (phenobarbital, theophylline or vitamin C) can lower bilirubin levels.

The normal range for the total bilirubin is 0.3 to 1.0 mg/dL and the normal level for direct bilirubin is 0.1 to 0.3 mg/dL. Indirect bilirubin levels range from 0.2 to 0.7 mg/dL. Neonates can have much larger total bilirubin levels, most of which is indirect bilirubin. High levels of bilirubin can also be seen in Gilbert syndrome, pancreatic cancer, gallbladder disease, transfusion reactions, and sickle cell anemia. Newborns should have total bilirubin levels of less than 10 mg/dL.

Hepatitis A

Hepatitis A is a viral liver infection transmitted by contaminated food or water. The test for hepatitis A is called the HAV test and will be positive even if you never had the infection but instead had the vaccine. IgM anti-HAV antibodies will be elevated in cases of acute infection and is able to be detected from two weeks up to twelve months following the contamination. IgG anti-HAV is a test that, when elevated, indicates an infection in the distant past. It begins to be elevated between 8-12 weeks following the onset of the infection. To evaluate whether or not the antibody elevation is due to acute infection or to the vaccination, check for liver function studies, which will be elevated in acute infection but not if the patient receives the vaccine. The test returns after about a week and is designated as positive or negative, depending on whether or not the infection has occurred or the patient has received the vaccination.

The test does not indicate whether or not the patient is infective as it only measures the antibodies to hepatitis A and not the active HAV particles.

Hepatitis B

Hepatitis B is a viral liver infection that is passed through the blood or bodily secretions. There are several hepatitis B tests used to identify the presence or absence of hepatitis B. HBV antibody testing can tell if the patient has had an infection. Ig M antibodies indicate an acute infection and IgG antibodies indicate an infection has occurred any time in the distant past.

HBsAg stands for "hepatitis B surface antigen" and indicates an acute transmissible infection or a chronic case of active hepatitis B. The test to show the clearance of the infection (anti-HBV) is positive about four weeks after the clearance of HBsAg from the bloodstream. If the person has a positive hepatitis B antibody test, they do not require an immunization against Hepatitis B.

Hepatitis B e-antigen, also known as HBeAg, will be positive in an acute infection. A hepatitis B DNA test will tell how much HepB DNA is in the blood and is a test to see if the treatment for hepatitis B is working. Hepatitis B core antibody or HBcAb is the test used to check blood that is slated to be transfused to see if it is safe to give. Hepatitis B e-antibody positivity indicates a near resolution of the hepatitis B infection. Immunization against hepatitis B is available and also prevents a person from getting hepatitis D, which only infects livers infected with hepatitis B first. All tests of antigens and antibodies are reported as "positive" or "negative".

Chapter 4: Arterial Blood Gases

Arterial blood gases are usually done under critical conditions when there is an issue regarding the ability of the lungs to exchange oxygen and carbon dioxide. The test also determines the acid-base balance in the system by measuring the pH of the blood. Arterial blood gases are a good way of identifying the severity of respiratory and metabolic disorders.

The two main blood gases are oxygen and carbon dioxide. In some situations, such as carbon monoxide poisoning, carbon monoxide can be found in higher than acceptable levels in the blood. Blood pH is measured by a special machine and is normally between 7.35 and 7.45. pH levels less than 7.35 indicate that the blood is too acidic; pH levels of greater than 7.45 indicate that the blood is too basic. The body uses bicarbonate (HCO_3^-) to adjust the pH of the blood. If the blood pH is too acidic, the kidneys increase the pH by increasing the concentration of the blood bicarbonate levels.

In an arterial blood gas measurement, the partial pressure of oxygen (PaO2) and the partial pressure of carbon dioxide (PaCO2) are measured along with the percent oxygen saturation. The blood pH is determined along with the bicarbonate level. The test measures the ability of the lungs to exchange oxygen for carbon dioxide and whether or not there is a metabolic or respiratory acidosis or alkalosis going on.

The normal values are as such:
·   PaO2: 75-100 mm Hg

·   PaCO2: 34-45 mm Hg

·   O2 saturation: 95-100 percent

·   Blood pH: 7.35-7.45

·   Bicarbonate: 20-29 mEq/L

If the pH is too low, the patient has either respiratory or metabolic acidosis. If the pH is too high, the patient has either respiratory or metabolic alkalosis. Blood gases are done in serious cases of chronic obstructive pulmonary disease (COPD), sepsis, kidney failure, pulmonary edema, Cushing disease, diabetes or drug overdose. All of these can yield a high bicarbonate level.

If the bicarbonate level is too low, it could indicate an overdose of alcohol, liver disease, aspirin overdose, dehydration, severe malnutrition, diarrhea, hyperventilation, kidney disease, shock, severe burns, and hyperthyroidism.

Blood consists of three different forms of carbon dioxide. They include bicarbonate HCO^{3-}, dissolved CO_2, and carbonic acid (H_2CO_3). Most of the carbon dioxide is in the form of HCO^{3-}ions. The blood gas level measures all forms of carbon dioxide at the same time. The total carbon dioxide level is normally 23-29 mmol/L in adults and 20-28 mmol/L in children. Elevated levels of total CO2 include pneumonia causing respiratory acidosis, COPD causing respiratory acidosis, Conn syndrome causing metabolic acidosis, Cushing syndrome causing metabolic acidosis, and alcoholism causing metabolic acidosis. Low levels of total CO2 are found in hyperventilation (respiratory alkalosis), cirrhosis (respiratory alkalosis), pneumonia (respiratory alkalosis), liver failure (respiratory alkalosis), diabetes (metabolic alkalosis), diarrhea (metabolic alkalosis), aspirin overdose (metabolic alkalosis), kidney failure (metabolic alkalosis), heart failure (metabolic alkalosis), antifreeze ingestion (metabolic alkalosis), methanol ingestion (metabolic alkalosis), and chronic starvation causing metabolic alkalosis.

Carbon monoxide binds to the hemoglobin cell, displacing oxygen by creating a complex called carboxyhemoglobin. This decreases the amount of oxygen capable of attaching to hemoglobin which can lead to death. Patients with excessive carbon monoxide poisoning will suffer from dizziness, visual disturbances, headache, confusion, muscle weakness, sleepiness, nausea and vomiting.

Chapter 5: Hematology Testing

Hematology testing involves testing of the red cells, white blood cells, and platelets in the body. Parameters of the red blood cells such as size and hemoglobin concentration red blood cells are included in a basic CBC (complete blood count) as these can aid in the diagnosis of blood diseases. Iron studies are included with basic hematology testing because many cases of anemia are caused by low iron. Coagulation studies are also a part of hematology testing and measure the degree of coagulation of the blood.

Hemoglobin

The hemoglobin molecule is the molecule contained inside red blood cells that carry oxygen from the lungs through the bloodstream to the cellular tissue and carries CO_2 from the cells back to the lungs. It is actually a complex of four large proteins that are bound together. There are alpha chains, beta chains and gamma chains. Two alpha hemoglobin chains combine with 2 beta hemoglobin chains to form the hemoglobin complex, while in fetuses and infants, there are mainly alpha chains connected to gamma chains, changing over to adult hemoglobin forms as the infant grows.

Iron is imbedded into the hemoglobin molecule and is essential for the holding on of oxygen and carbon dioxide. Hemoglobin is responsible for the natural donut-shaped shape of the red blood cell. With abnormalities of the hemoglobin molecule, such as seen in sickle cell anemia, the shape of the red blood cell changes.

The normal hemoglobin range in individuals varies with age. For example, a newborn hemoglobin level is 17-22 gm/dL. This rapidly returns to the childhood levels over one month to become a normal range of 11-13 gm/dL. Adult females have hemoglobin levels of between 12 and 16 gm/dL while in males the normal range is 14-18 gm/dL.

Low hemoglobin levels are referred to as anemia, while high hemoglobin levels can be seen in diseases such as polycythemia vera.

Hematocrit

The hematocrit is a measure of the percentage of blood cells that encompass red blood cells. The normal range is 38.8-50 percent in men and 34.9-44.5 percent in women. Children have somewhat different hematocrit levels depending on age with normal levels coming by the age of 15 years in both men and women. The hemoglobin and hematocrit levels often go up and down together.

Mean Corpuscular Volume (MCV)

The MCV is a measure of the average size/volume of the red cells in the body. A low MCV is indicative of a microcytic condition and a high MCV is indicative of a macrocytic condition. The normal value is 80-96 fL/red cells in adults. The reference range varies somewhat depending on age. The MCV is used along with the MCH (mean corpuscular hemoglobin level) and the MCHC (mean corpuscular hemoglobin concentration) in order to determine what type of anemia is going on. Another test, called the RDW or "red cell distribution" is included and is a measure of the difference between the smallest red blood cells and the largest red blood cells or a measure of the variability in red blood cell size.

Microcytic anemia usually means the patient has iron deficiency anemia, thalassemia, anemia of chronic disease or sideroblastic anemia. Macrocytic anemia is usually caused by vitamin B12 or folate deficiency, hemolytic anemia, liver disease, alcoholism, hypothyroidism, aplastic anemia, or myelodysplastic syndrome.

There are certain types of anemia that have normal-sized rbcs. These include anemia from acute blood loss, anemia of chronic disease, hemolytic anemias, anemia of kidney disease and aplastic anemia.

Mean Corpuscular Hemoglobin (MCH)

This is the amount of hemoglobin per cell on average. In adults, this value is 27-33 pg/cell. It is closely related to the MCHC as they both reveal the amount of hemoglobin in the cells. All three parameters, MCV, MCH and MCHC are important in telling what type of anemia a person has. Nowadays, since the RDW became available, it, along with the MCV are primarily used in defining what kind of anemia a person has.

White Blood Cell Count (WBC)

White blood cells are our infection fighting cells and are together known as the "leukocytes". The five major types of WBCs include these:

1. Neutrophils

2. Lymphocytes

3. Monocytes

4. Eosinophils

5. Basophils

A normal WBC count is 4,500 to 10,000 wbc/mcL. Many machines will perform manual differential, which says the percentage of each type of WBC there is. Elevated neutrophil counts usually indicate bacterial infections are present, while elevated lymphocyte counts usually mean that a viral infection is present; however, none of this is hard and fast. You can also ask for a manual count in which the lab technician counts the percentage of each type of WBC is found on a slide drawn from the vial of blood.

Low WBC counts are called leukopenia. A total WBC count less than 4,500 means leukopenia is present. The risk of infection goes up if the WBC count is very low, such as less than 500 neutrophils per microliter of blood. Leukopenia is caused by:

1.Chemotherapy

2.Bone marrow insufficiency or failure

3.Autoimmune diseases

4.Radiation therapy

5.Liver or spleen diseases

6.Bone marrow cancers

7.Viral infections such as infectious mononucleosis

8.Very dangerous bacterial infections

9.Medications like antibiotics, anti-thyroid drugs, seizure medications, captopril, diuretics, clozapine, chlorpromazine, sulfonamides, H2 blockers, ticlopidine, terbinafine and quinidine

A high WBC count is called leukocytosis. Leukocytosis is due to the following:

2. Medications such as Beta agonists, steroids, epinephrine, heparin, and lithium

3. Anemia

4. Smoking

5. Bacterial infections

6. Inflammatory diseases

7. Leukemia

8. Severe physical or emotional stress

9. Severe tissue damage such as is seen in burns

10. Having had a splenectomy

Platelets

Platelets help the blood clot. They are small cells that do not have a nucleus. A normal platelet count is 150,000 to 400,000 platelets per mcL.

The platelet count can be low without a high risk of bleeding. You won't have a higher than normal risk of bleeding until the platelet count is less than 50,000. This condition is known as thrombocytopenia. It can be due to not enough platelets being made inside the bone marrow, increased destruction of the platelets in the bloodstream, or increased destruction of platelets in the liver or spleen. Causes of low platelet counts include certain medications, chemotherapy, radiation, and autoimmune disorders.

A high platelet count (greater than 400,000) is called thrombocytosis and occurs in certain types of anemia, certain medications, cancer, chronic myelogenous leukemia, polycythemia vera, recent splenic removal, certain infections, or primary thrombocythemia.

The normal platelet volume is 7.2-11.7 fL. If the mean platelet volume or MPV is beyond this normal range, the patient should be assessed for blocked vessel disease.

Prothrombin Time (PT or Protime)

The protime is just one measure of the time it takes to clot blood. It is measured to check for bleeding disorders and to measure the effectiveness of blood clotting drugs such as warfarin. The protime has been standardized and is now called the INR, which stands for international normalizing ration. The INR is a standardized method of determining blood clotting that doesn't vary according to how the test was done. Prothrombin is also called factor II clotting factor. The protime assesses the function of the clotting factors I, II, V, VII, and X.

A long protime is due to warfarin, low levels of clotting factors, low activity of the clotting factors, clotting factor inhibitors, liver disease, and an increased use of the clotting factors. It is assessed whenever there is suspicion of a clotting disorder, such as hemophilia, to check for low vitamin K levels, before surgery, and to see if the liver is working properly.

A normal protime is between 11 and 13 seconds with an INR of 0.8 to 1.1. An acceptable INR for a person on Coumadin (warfarin) is between 2 and 3.

Partial thromboplastin time (PTT)

This is another test of the ability of the blood to clot. It is usually used to test for the effectiveness of heparin on the bleeding time. The Protime and the PTT are often assessed together. A normal PTT is between 30 and 40 seconds. A person on heparin should have a PTT that is between 1.5 and 2.5 seconds longer than normal.

DIC or disseminated intravascular coagulation is a severe disorder in which excessive clotting has used up all the clotting factors so that bleeding occurs. This disorder can be life-threatening. Long

PTTs can also be seen in cases of factor XII deficiency, lupus anticoagulant syndrome, antiphospholipid antibody syndrome, nephrotic syndrome, heparin use, or hypofibrinogenemia.

Ferritin

This is a measure of the iron stores of the body. It is found in iron-storing cells for use when needed. A normal range for males is 12-300 ng/mL and a normal range for females is 12-150 ng/mL. The lower the amount of ferritin in the blood, the lesser is the amount of iron stores in the body.

A high ferritin level is often due to frequent blood transfusions, alcoholic liver disease, or hemochromatosis. Low levels of ferritin are found in heavy menstrual bleeding, chronic digestive tract bleeding, and poor absorption of iron due to intestinal problems.

Total Iron Binding Capacity (TIBC)

This is a measure that, along with the serum iron test, helps determine if the patient has iron deficiency or iron overload. The normal TIBC is about 20-40 percent of total transferrin sites used to transport iron. It is a measure of the amount of transferrin loaded with iron. In iron deficiency anemia, the total iron is low but the TIBC is increased to try and hold onto as much iron as possible and the transferrin saturation is low. In hemochromatosis, the serum iron level is high but the TIBC will be low to normal with an increase in transferrin saturation. Transferrin levels will be low in liver disease because it is the liver that makes transferrin for the body.

Serum Iron

The serum iron level is the level of iron in the bloodstream. It is used along with the TIBC, percent transferrin saturation and Ferritin level to determine what kind of anemia a person has. For example, in iron deficiency anemia, the iron level is low, the TIBC is high, the percent transferrin saturation is low and the ferritin level is low. The normal serum iron level is 60-170 mcg/dL.

Chapter 6: Cardiovascular Testing

Whenever there are symptoms of a heart attack, with or without the presence of EKG changes, cardiac testing may be performed to see if there is laboratory evidence for damage to the heart. Whenever the heart is damaged, the cells release cardiac enzymes that can be detected in the bloodstream. These tests can be invaluable in the detection and management of a heart attack. Generally, the greater the elevation in cardiac enzymes, the greater is the area of heart damage during a heart attack.

Troponin

Troponin can be broken up into three separate regulatory proteins, such as troponin C, troponin I, and Troponin T. These proteins can be found in skeletal muscle and in cardiac muscle but is not found in smooth muscle. The test for troponin measures the levels of troponin I and troponin T within the bloodstream. High levels of troponin indicate a recent heart attack. It is usually released soon after the heart attack and dissipates over a period of 7-14 days following a heart attack. It is a test often used alongside a CPK test, described below.

Other causes of an increased troponin level include having a rapid heart rate, pulmonary hypertension, pulmonary embolism, congestive heart failure, myocarditis, extreme exercise, trauma to the heart, chronic kidney disease or cardiomyopathy. The troponin levels can increase following coronary angioplasty with stenting, defibrillation, open heart surgery, and radiofrequency ablation involving heart muscle.

Creatinine Phosphokinase (CPK) Test

Creatinine phosphokinase is a cellular enzyme found in the brain, heart, and skeletal muscle. It can be increased in situations of a heart attack. CPK isoenzymes are often done along with the CPK test to tell if the CPK elevation is due to heart damage or damage to the brain or skeletal muscle.

Certain medications will raise the CPK level, including some anesthetics, amphotericin B, fibrates, statins, cocaine, alcohol, and dexamethasone. People who have dermatomyositis, polymyositis or severe skeletal muscle damage will have elevations of the CPK. The normal value of CPK is between 10 and 120 mcg/L.

Elevations in CPK can be seen in seizure disorders, strokes, delirium tremens, pulmonary infarction, electric shock, heart attack, myopathies, rhabdomyalysis, and low or high thyroid conditions. CPK levels rise when a heart attack occurs but dissipate within 48 hours. Isoenzymes of CPK include the following:

· CPK-1: from the brain and lungs

· CPK-2: from the heart

· CPK-3: from the skeletal muscle

When a CPK is found to be elevated, CPK isoenzymes can be done to determine the exact source of the CPK.

Lactate Dehydrogenase (LDH)

The LDH is an enzyme found in several body tissues, including the liver, heart, muscles, brain, lungs and red blood cells. Whenever there is tissue damage to any of these areas, there will be elevations of the LDH. LDH isoenzymes can tell the source of the elevation when the test is elevated.

Drugs that can elevate the LDH level include narcotic medications, mithramycin, fluorides, clofibrate, aspirin, anesthetics, and procainamide. Anemia and leukemia can increase the level of LDH in the bloodstream as well. A normal value for LDH is 105-333 IU/L.

The LDH can be elevated in a heart attack as well as in situations involving infectious mononucleosis, hemolytic anemia, liver disease, muscle injury, low blood pressure, muscular dystrophy, pancreatitis, cancer, tissue death or stroke.

There are five different isoenzymes of LDH and ordering isoenzymes may be done to identify the source of the elevated value.

· LDH-1 is found in heart muscle and in red blood cells

· LDH-2 is found in WBCs

· LDH-3 is found in the lung

- LDH-4 is concentrated in the placenta, the pancreas, and in the kidneys

- LDH-5 is concentrated in the liver and skeletal muscle

The LDH is elevated shortly after a heart attack and returns to normal within 10-14 days.

Aspartate Transaminase (AST)

This was the first cardiac enzyme identified for detection of heart attack. It is not very specific for a heart attack, however, as it is used to identify liver dysfunction as well.

It is best to check all the cardiac proteins and enzymes, including the isoenzymes, in order to make sense out of the blood tests which may or may not individually represent a heart attack.

Brain Natriuretic Peptide (BNP)

BNP is a protein that is released from the heart whenever the heart must do excessive amounts of work as is seen in heart failure. It is therefore used as a laboratory confirmation of a suspected case of heart failure. Another test is called the N-terminal pro-brain natriuretic peptide or NT-proBNP. The test is ideally done on a fasting basis and is affected by cardiac glycoside and diuretic use. People on dialysis or who have COPD will have elevated levels of BNP. Some herbal supplements, such as Echinacea or valerian root can adversely affect the test. The normal range for the BNP is 0-99 pg/ml. The higher the level, up to a range of about 900 pg/ml will be indicative of heart failure. It can indicate heart failure with or without the presence of an acute myocardial infarction.

Chapter 7: Endocrine Tests

The endocrine system involves a wide range of hormones sent from many glands throughout the body. Laboratory testing can help determine if a particular gland is overworking or underworking. Many hormone systems have a feedback loop that must be intact in order to have the hormone levels remain normal.

CRH and ACTH

The hypothalamus in the brain produces and releases corticotropin-releasing hormone (CRH) which triggers the pituitary gland to release ACTH, also called adrenocorticotropic hormone. This, in turn, triggers the release of cortisol from the adrenal glands, raising glucose and blood pressure while suppressing the immune system. As cortisol levels go up, ACTH levels fall. Cortisol peaks in the morning and is at a trough level by evening. Therefore, it is important to determine the time when the cortisol level is to be taken from the patient's veins. Peak levels are done between 6 am and 8 am, while trough levels are done between 6 pm and 11 pm. It is necessary to put the blood on ice as soon as it is gotten from the patient and the test must be done as soon as possible. Things like lithium, insulin and amphetamines may increase the cortisol levels.

The normal range for ACTH at 6 am to 8 am is less than 80 pg/ml. The normal level for ACTH at 6 pm to 11 pm is less than 50 pg/ml. The normal peak ranges for cortisol are 5-23 mcg/dL and the normal trough ranges are 3-13 mcg/dL.

Elevated cortisol levels are found in physical or emotional distress, Cushing's disease, Adrenal gland tumor, pituitary gland tumor. Low levels of cortisol can be seen in a stroke, head injury, pituitary gland tumor, adrenal gland tumor or pituitary radiation.

Comparisons are made between the ACTH and cortisol levels. For example, if the ACTH and cortisol levels are both high, then ACTH is being made outside the pituitary gland. If there are low levels of ACTH and high levels of cortisol, this can be caused by Cushing syndrome. High ACTH and low cortisol levels are found in Addison's disease. Low levels of both ACTH and cortisol are found in situations of hypopituitarism.

Dexamethasone Suppression Test

This is a test for Cushing's syndrome. Dexamethasone mimics cortisol in the blood and is given at 11 pm the night before the cortisol level is taken (at about 8 am). Some people metabolize dexamethasone quickly so that increased amounts of dexamethasone must be given if Cushing's disease is suspected but the results were suboptimal. Ideally, the cortisol level should be very low after receiving dexamethasone and, if it is not, there may be an adrenal gland tumor secreting cortisol in spite of low ACTH levels. The patient may receive up to 8 separate doses of dexamethasone over a two day period of time. In a normal dexamethasone suppression test, the cortisol level will be less than 5 mcg/dL. High levels can also be seen in uncontrolled diabetes, elevated thyroid syndromes, heart attacks, heart failure, poor diet, alcoholism, depression, anorexia, fever, or lung cancer.

Another test of cortisol that is not time-dependent is the 24 hour urine free cortisol test. The test is negatively impacted by the taking of lithium, MAOIs, morphine, barbiturates, birth control pills, Dilantin, aspirin, methadone, Aldactone or diuretics.

Aldosterone Level

Aldosterone is secreted by the adrenal gland to cause the kidneys to release renin, which raises blood pressure. Aldosterone also causes an increase in the sodium and fluid volume of the blood. Aldosterone and renin activity are usually measured at the same time. Aldosterone can be measured as the 24 hour urine excretion of aldosterone and can detect an overactive adrenal gland. High levels of aldosterone can be due to an adrenal gland tumor. Eating natural black licorice is prohibited for two weeks before the test. The person needs to eat a 3 gram per day sodium diet (normal sodium diet) for two weeks before the test because low and high sodium diets can adversely affect the test. The patient's positioning, such as lying, standing or sitting can affect the aldosterone levels. If the patient stands or sits for two hours prior to the test, this will raise aldosterone levels.

Medications such as estrogen, diuretics, corticosteroids, opiates, NSAIDs, progesterone, heparin and Aldactone can adversely affect the test. Aldosterone levels are increased with stress and decrease with age. The normal aldosterone level when the patient has been lying down is 3-10 ng/dL. The normal level for sitting or standing patients is 5-30 ng/dL. If the level is high, this could mean adrenal hyperplasia or Conn syndrome.

Cortisol

The cortisol level is highest in the morning and lowest at night but these numbers reverse themselves whenever a person works nights and sleeps during the day. Low cortisol levels signal ACTH to be released by the pituitary gland. The cortisol level can be drawn as a part of a dexamethasone suppression test, an ACTH test or a 24 hour urine collection test. For the blood test, the person should lie down for thirty minutes prior to the test in order to reduce stress levels in the patient. Pregnancy can increase cortisol levels. Normal morning levels of cortisol are 5-23 mcg/dL. Normal afternoon levels are 3-13 mcg/dL.

Elevated levels of cortisol are seen in Cushing's syndrome, adrenal gland tumor or an overactive adrenal gland, severe liver disease, depression, elevated thyroxine levels, obesity, kidney disease, and sepsis. Low cortisol levels are seen in Addison's disease, Sheehan syndrome, shock, and autoimmune diseases.

Estrogen

There are three types of estrogen, which is produced by the ovaries, muscles, fatty tissue, placenta, testicles and adrenal glands. The three types of estrogen are estradiol, Estriol, and estrone. Estriol is mainly produced by the placenta after the ninth week of pregnancy. Estrogen levels are measured in people who are likely to have ovarian or testicular cancer, or an adrenal gland tumor. Estrone is produced primarily in postmenopausal women. Medications that can interfere with the test include Clomid and prednisone. Normal estradiol levels before menopause are 30-400 ng/ml. Normal estradiol levels after menopause are less than 30 ng/ml. Men have estradiol levels of 10-50 pg/ml.

Elevated estrogen levels are seen in ovarian cancer, multiple fetuses in pregnancy, cirrhosis, successful infertility treatment, early puberty, testicular cancer, or an adrenal gland tumor. Low estrogen levels are seen in Turner syndrome, anorexia, and poor pituitary gland function.

Growth Hormone

Growth hormone is secreted by the pituitary gland and stimulates the growth of cells, reproduction and the levels of insulin-like growth factor-1. Just the IGF-1 test might be drawn, the growth hormone stimulating test using insulin, or the growth hormone suppression test may be drawn. It is checked when there is a suspicion of a growth hormone tumor in the pituitary gland. The taking of insulin, estrogen, St. John's Wort, amphetamines, birth control pills, and steroids can adversely affect the test. The normal growth hormone level in men is less than 5 ng/ml and in women is less than 10 ng/ml. Elevated GH levels are seen in gigantism, acromegaly, starvation, kidney disease, diabetes or a pituitary gland tumor.

Luteinizing Hormone

LH is produced by the pituitary gland and stimulates both testosterone production and ovulation in women. It is the chemical used in ovulation predictor kits. It is a test for infertility assessment or to see if there is an underlying cause of irregular menstrual periods. It can be seen in menopause, precocious puberty or delayed puberty and erectile dysfunction. Medications such as digitalis, spironolactone, anti-seizure medication, naloxone, levodopa or clomiphene, cimetidine, phenothiazine, and birth control pills can affect the test.

The LH levels in the follicular phase of the cycle is 1-18 IU/L; midcycle phase is 8.7-80 IU/L; luteal phase 0.5-18 IU/L. Women after menopause have LH levels of 12-55 IU/L and men have LH levels of 1-9 IU/L.

High levels of LH are seen in polycystic ovarian syndrome, absence of ovaries, early puberty, Klinefelter syndrome (in men) or the absence/malfunction of the testicles. A poorly functioning pituitary gland may lead to low LH levels. Other causes of low LH include anorexia, a poorly functioning hypothalamus, and low body weight.

Parathyroid Hormone

Parathyroid hormone is made by four parathyroid glands imbedded in the thyroid gland. It is released in response to low calcium levels, allowing for more retention of calcium by the kidneys and more release of calcium by the bones. PTH allows for the conversion of vitamin D to an active form increasing calcium absorption by the gut. Calcium and phosphorus levels are often drawn along with the PTH level. Calcium and phosphorus have an inverse relationship in the bloodstream. The test should be done in the morning when the patient is fasting. Cimetidine, Inderal or Betachron ER will lower the test result. Lithium, rifampin, diuretics, Lasix, thiazide diuretics, and anti-seizure medication can raise the PTH levels.

The normal level for PTH is 10-65 pg/ml. High PTH levels are seen in parathyroid tumors, low calcium levels, pancreatic cancer, renal disease, lung cancer, malabsorption syndromes, ovarian cancer or vitamin D deficiency. Low PTH levels are seen in low Mg levels, high calcium intake, lymphoma, poorly functioning parathyroid glands, multiple myeloma or sarcoidosis.

Thyroid Testing

The hypothalamus releases TRH (thyrotropin-releasing hormone), which stimulates the pituitary gland to release TSH (thyroid stimulating hormone. This causes the thyroid gland to release thyroxine (T4) and triiodothyronine (T3). The production of T4 and T3 depend on the iodine concentration of the blood. T4 and T3 are mostly transported by thyroid binding globulin in the bloodstream and there is much less unbound T4 and T3. The four main thyroid tests performed are:

- Total T4

- Free T4

- Free thyroxine index (FTI)

- T3 test

The TSH level is reciprocal to the T4 and T3 levels. Therefore, the TSH level is usually high in primary hypothyroidism. The TSH is low in primary hyperthyroidism or because of a pituitary insufficiency.

Things that adversely affect the tests include the taking of corticosteroids, Dilantin, Tegretol, warfarin, heparin, aspirin, lithium, propranolol, amiodarone, estrogen, progesterone or birth control pills. Normal values of total thyroxine are 5-14 mcg/dL in adults; for the total T3 is 80-230 ng/dL; for the free T3 is 0.2-0.6

ng/dL. Elevated levels of T4 and T3 are seen in elevated thyroid diseases, Grave's disease, thyroiditis, goiter, or an overdose of thyroid medications. Low levels of T4 and T3 are seen in low thyroid conditions, thyroid radiation, or pituitary insufficiency. Normal TSH values in adults are 0.4-4.5 mIU/L. Elevated TSH levels are seen in low thyroid conditions, pituitary gland tumors, and Hashimoto thyroiditis. Low levels of TSH are seen in elevated thyroid conditions, goiter, toxic nodule tumor, pituitary gland insufficiency, and Grave's disease.

Testosterone

Testosterone is stimulated by the release of LH from the pituitary gland and is made by the adrenal glands, ovaries and testes. Testosterone is bound to sex hormone-binding globulin (SHBG) or is free in the bloodstream. The test is thrown off if the person is taking birth control pills, Aldactone, testosterone, digoxin, corticosteroids, barbiturates, estrogen, or some seizure medication. People with an elevated or low thyroid condition will have problems taking an accurate testosterone level.

Normal levels of testosterone in males are 280-1080 ng/dL above the age of 19. Normal levels of testosterone in women are less than 70 ng/dL above the age of 16. Elevated levels of testosterone are seen in testicular cancer, ovarian cancer, or adrenal gland cancer, polycystic ovarian syndrome or precocious puberty. Low levels are seen in Klinefelter syndrome in males, cirrhosis, testicular disorders, and alcoholism. Pituitary gland disorders can cause low testosterone.

Chapter 8: Pregnancy and Genetic Testing

These are tests used to detect causes of infertility, to detect the presence of pregnancy and to look for possible genetic causes of birth defects. They are done on women and children, depending on the test.

Anti-sperm Antibody Test

This is a test that is used for infertility. Women can make antibodies against male semen, killing the sperm before they can fertilize the egg. The antibodies can be found in vaginal fluids, semen or blood. Men can have a positive anti-sperm antibody test if he has had a prostate gland infection, a testicular injury, or a vasectomy. Women, too, can develop anti-sperm antibodies from her partner's sperm. In women, the test is simply a blood test. In males, the test is done on semen in which ejaculation has not taken place within 2 days of the test. The ejaculate must reach the laboratory within 30 minutes of collection through masturbation into a sterile cup. The test is reported as positive or negative, depending on whether or not anti-sperm antibodies are found.

Alpha-fetoprotein or AFP

This is a protein made by the fetal liver. The AFP level rises at around 14 weeks gestation, reaching a peak at 34 weeks gestation. It is used to detect the presence of possible birth defects in the fetus. It is part of a maternal serum triple screen which also detects the amount of beta-HCG and estrogen in the maternal blood. A quadruple screen can also be done, which adds the level of the hormone inhibin A to the triple screen.

AFP can also be detected in anyone with the following diseases: Hodgkin disease, lymphoma, testicular cancer, ovarian cancer, pancreatic cancer, and renal cell cancer. Not all of these cancers will demonstrate elevations in alpha-fetoprotein.

In pregnant women, the test is done between 15 and 20 weeks gestation. Normal values depend on the gestational age and weight of the pregnant person. AFP levels are higher in African-Americans and lower in Asian women. The AFT level is elevated in trisomy 18, Down syndrome, anencephaly, omphalocele, spina bifida or hepatoma (in those who have chronic cirrhosis or hepatitis B).

Smoking and insulin-dependency can increase the levels of AFP in the blood. Elevated AFP levels in pregnancy indicate the need for an ultrasound and/or an amniocentesis. Normal levels of AFP I a woman 12-22 weeks gestation are 19-75 IU/ml. In non-pregnant individuals, the AFP level is 0-6.4 IU/ml. High levels in pregnancy can mean multiple fetuses, a dead fetus or an incorrectly calculated gestational age. Low levels in pregnancy can mean Down syndrome with an accuracy of 60 percent. When the AFP is done as part of a triple screen, the accuracy increases to 80 percent. A normal AFP does not mean that Down syndrome is not present.

Follicle Stimulating Hormone

This is a hormone made by the pituitary gland by men and women. It controls egg and sperm production. It is a constant value in men but rises and falls with the menstrual cycle in women. The highest level of FSH in women is at the time of ovulation. LH, estrogen, and progesterone levels are sometimes ordered along with the FSH in women to get a complete picture of the hormonal milieu.

Normal FSH levels in women: follicular phase 5-20 IU/L. Peak at midcycle 30-50 IU/L. Luteal phase 5-20 IU/L. After menopause, the FSH level is higher than 49 IU/L. Men have FSH levels of 5-15 IU/L. Elevated FSH levels are seen in polycystic ovarian syndrome, ovarian failure, menopause, abnormal testicular function, Klinefelter syndrome (in men), children, and the beginning of puberty. Low FSH levels are seen in lack of ovulation, lack of sperm, malnutrition, hypothalamic disorder, pituitary gland dysfunction, and stress.

Human Chorionic Gonadotropin (HCG)

HCG is produced by the placenta. It is detectable at the time of missed menstrual period (and sometimes as early as five days before) in pregnant women. The level increases to a peak at 16 weeks gestation and decreases to zero at the time of birth. It is detected by urine and blood samples. In blood samples, a quantitative HCG can be determined. HCG is also part of the triple screen done in pregnant women. HCG can be elevated in non-pregnant women who have a molar pregnancy, uterine cancer, ovarian cancer and other types of tumors. Testicular cancer can yield elevated HCG levels in men.

Normal levels of HCG in men are less than 5 IU/L. In pregnant women 24-28 days' gestation, the level is 5-100 IU/L. At 4-5 weeks gestation, the level is 50-500 IU/L. Levels reach a peak of around 270,000 IU/L. High levels in men can be seen in pancreatic cancer, colon cancer, lung cancer, liver cancer, uterine cancer, and ovarian cancer. In women, high levels can be seen in multiple fetuses, Down syndrome or molar pregnancy. Low HCG levels in women who are pregnant can mean an ectopic pregnancy or a miscarriage.

Inhibin A

This is secreted by the placenta and is part of the quadruple screen in pregnancy. It is checked around 20 weeks gestation to check for birth defects such as Down syndrome. High inhibin A levels are seen in birth defects. Additional tests must be done if the patient has an elevated level.

Prolactin

Prolactin is produced by the pituitary gland during pregnancy and lactation. Ejection of milk is inhibited by progesterone during pregnancy and is allowed to eject after progesterone levels fall following pregnancy. Suckling stimulates prolactin release. Prolactin levels are higher in the morning. Normal prolactin levels are 20-400 ng/ml in pregnant women. In non-pregnant women, the level is less than 25 ng/ml. In men, the normal level is less than 20 ng/ml. It is used to check for prolactinoma of the pituitary gland, to check for a cause of infertility, to check to see why there is nipple discharge, and to check for erectile dysfunction in men.

Phenylketonuria Test (PKU test)

In phenylketonuria, an infant does not make phenylalanine hydroxylase—an enzyme that metabolizes phenylalanine into tyrosine. PKU is genetic and can be tested on a neonate between 12 and 28 hours following birth. It is sometimes repeated at one week of age. The test measures the level of phenylalanine hydroxylase in the newborn's blood. If an infant has phenylketonuria, he or she can suffer from mental retardation and a seizure disorder. This must be tested after the newborn has begun to drink formula or breast milk.

Tay-Sachs Test

Tay-Sachs disease is a genetic disease in which the infant does not have hexosaminidase A—an enzyme that metabolizes the fatty acid, ganglioside. Nerve damage can occur in a child with Tay-Sachs disease. The test measures the amount of hexosaminidase A in the blood of the newborn. It can be checked as part of a chorionic villus sampling or amniocentesis. The normal total hexosaminidase level is 10.4-23.8 U/L. Half of the normal result indicates a carrier of the disease. It may be tested as a part of testing for Sandhoff disease, in which the patient is missing both hexosaminidase A and B.

Sickle Cell Test

In sickle cell disease, the individual's red blood cells contain hemoglobin S, which causes the red blood cells to become sickle-shaped. It is an autosomal recessive disease found mainly in the African-American population. Infants younger than six months of age can have a negative result even if they have the disease. The test is done after the age of six months, when fetal hemoglobin has left the system. It can be tested as part of a chorionic villus sampling or as part of an amniocentesis. A patient can be heterozygous and possess the sickle cell trait or homozygous, having sickle cell disease. The test checks for the level of hemoglobin S in the red blood cells.

Hemochromatosis Test

This test checks for hemochromatosis, which involves an increase in iron absorption and iron stores in the body. A ferritin level can be tested to check for the disease or a DNA test for the presence of the hemochromatosis gene. The test is reported as positive if the HFE gene is mutated.

Chapter 9: Infection Testing

There are blood tests to check for various types of infection, including bacterial and viral blood testing. These are checked along with tests like a complete CBC to assess the patient for infection. There are also antibody tests that can tell if a person's immune system has been sensitized and has created antibodies against the particular substance.

Antibody Tests

Antibodies are simply proteins made by lymphocytes in the immune system against bacteria and other microorganisms designed to target the microorganism for killing by other cells in the immune system. Antibodies can also be made against red blood cells that do not match the receptors on the recipient's blood cells in a transfusion reaction. One test is the Rh antibody test. If the woman is Rh negative and her fetus is Rh positive, the mixing of the blood can cause the woman to fight off fetal tissue as if it were foreign tissue. An Rh antibody titer is done on pregnant women who are Rh negative to see if she has been sensitized against the Rh factor. Sensitization usually occurs when blood is mixed at the time of birth so Rh disease is usually only a problem of second and more pregnancies. Rhogam is given during subsequent pregnancies to block sensitivity.

Indirect Coomb's Test

This is a test to identify whether or not there has been the production of antibodies against red blood cells in a transfusion reaction. It is done on the recipient or donor red blood cells to see if the antibodies are in the blood sample. The test is negative or positive, depending on the presence of antibodies or not. A direct Coomb's test checks if there are RBC antibodies in the recipient's blood and an indirect Coomb's test checks to see if the donor blood is compatible with the recipient's blood. When an Rh-negative mother is sensitized, the indirect Coomb's test will be positive.

Blood Culture and Sensitivity

This is a test for bacteria in the bloodstream of an infected patient. Blood is taken under sterile conditions and is grown in a medium and on a culture dish. If bacteria grow, the bacterium species is identified. Small tabs of paper impregnated with antibiotics are set upon the culture dish and the dish is left to incubate for another day or so. If the antibiotic kills the bacteria, there is a zone of clearing around the disc to show that the bacteria could not grow in the presence of the infused antibiotic. The blood must be drawn at two different times from three different veins to make sure there is no contamination from skin bacteria during the blood draw. It can take between 3 and 10 days to get an accurate blood culture and sensitivity test. Fungal infections may be detected as late as 30 days from the blood draw.

Mononucleosis Tests

Mononucleosis is caused by the EBV (Epstein-Barr virus). The test for mononucleosis assesses the blood for antibodies to the EBV. A monospot test checks for heterophil antibodies which form between two and nine weeks post-infection. A false negative test can occur if the infection is newer than two weeks. A normal monospot test is "negative". A positive monospot can occur with mononucleosis infection, leukemia, rheumatoid arthritis, lymphoma, or hepatitis.

An EBV antibody titer can return in three days. The titer represents how much of the sample of blood needed to be diluted until the antibodies were no longer detected. The higher the ratio, the greater the number of EBV antibodies in the sample. A normal EBV titer is less than 1:40. The test can tell if the infection is acute or chronic. IgM antibodies are acute antibodies, meaning that there is an acute infection. IgG antibodies indicate that the infection has happened in the distant past.

Helicobacter pylori Tests

H. pylori is a type of bacterium that infects the duodenum and stomach, leading to peptic ulcers. Having H. pylori does not mean that you have an ulcer but that there is the potential for an ulcer. There are four different H. pylori tests. The first is the Helicobacter pylori antibody test, which checks if you have ever been infected with H. pylori. A urea breath test checks for the presence of H. pylori in the stomach. The H. pylori stool antigen test assesses whether or not there is active H. pylori antigens in the stool. A stomach biopsy can also detect the presence of an H. pylori infection. False negative tests are possible in all four situations.

The tests come back as positive or negative for the presence of H. pylori antigens or antibodies. The urea breath test is reported in three hours and is normal if there is no tagged hydrocarbon in the breath sample. The patient must take a radioactive, yet harmless, pill before taking the breath test. Medications for ulcers such as Carafate, Prilosec, Pepcid, Zantac and Aciphex can cause a false negative result.

Herpes Simplex Virus Tests

HSV or herpes simplex virus causes blisters and painful sores on the skin and mucus membranes in the mouth, throat, vagina, urethra, penis, and nose. There are two types: HSV-1, which is usually spread orally through the use of shared utensils or kissing someone who has a cold sore on their lips; and HSV-2, which is usually called genital herpes and is passed through sexual activity.

There are four HSV tests: 1) HSV antibody test, which checks for antibodies in the blood but cannot tell if it is HSV-1 or HSV-2. 2) PCR test or polymerase chain reaction test. This is a test that involves a cell scraping that can identify the difference between HSV-1 and HSV-2. 3) A herpes viral culture can detect the presence of HSV-2 in culture from a cell scraping. 4) Herpes virus antigen detection test, which can detect Herpes virus antigen under the microscope.

Lyme Disease

The Lyme disease tests for the presence of Borrelia burgdorferi bacterium which is transmitted from the bite of a deer tick. The test checks for the presence of B. burgdorferi antibodies in the blood. An indirect fluorescent antibody teste or IFA, an ELISA (enzyme-linked immunosorbent assay) and a Western blot test can be done. The Western blot test is the definitive test while the IFA and the ELISA are screening tests. There can be a false negative test if the infection happened within 2 months of the test date. False positive tests can occur if the B. burgdorferi infection has resolved and is past. The test results are reported as low, normal, or high. The test of the IFA is reported as a titer with normal being less than 1:256. The ELISA is reported as negative or positive. The Western blot test is reported as positive or negative for B. burgdorferi antibodies.

Rubella Test

Rubella is also called German measles and can cause congenital rubella syndrome if a pregnant woman has the infection while pregnant. It is checked on the first obstetrical visit on every patient. The test checks for the presence of rubella virus antibodies in the system. IgG antibodies indicate a distant past infection, while IgM antibodies are present in an acute or recent infection. IgG antibodies can be present because of a past infection or immunization involving rubella. A negative IgG antibody test in a pregnant woman means she must avoid being around anyone at risk or suspected of having German measles. Ideally, a woman should be immunized against rubella at least a month before becoming pregnant.

Syphilis Testing

Syphilis is an infection involving the Treponema pallidum bacterium. There are seven different syphilis tests:

1. VDRL—checks for anticardiolipin antibodies in a patient who has syphilis. It is a screening test for syphilis.

2. RPR (rapid plasma regain)—this is an antibody test for syphilis that doesn't require a microscope.

3. ELISA—detects the presence of T. pallidum antibodies as a screening test for syphilis.

4. FTA-ABS—this is the fluorescent treponemal antibody absorption test that is positive about 4 weeks of an infection.

5. TPPA—this is the Treponema pallidum partial agglutination assay, which does not test spinal fluid as is done in the FTA-ABS test.

6. Dark Field Microscopy—this identifies the T. pallidum under a dark field microscope.

7. Microhemoagglutination assay (MHA-TP)—this is like the TPPA test.

A positive VDRL or RPR does not definitely mean that the patient has syphilis. The FTA-ABS, TPPA, and MHA-TP tests are positive even after the infection has resolved. Samples for these tests can be done on blood or on spinal fluid

A normal test is a nonreactive antibody test with no T. pallidum seen under dark field microscope. An inconclusive test is when the antibody is detected but there are no T. pallidum under the microscope. A positive test for an active infection is when the T. pallidum is seen under dark field microscope of cerebrospinal fluid or blood.

Chapter 10: Lipid and Pancreatic Testing

The pancreas is an exocrine and endocrine organ that produces digestive enzymes as well as the hormones insulin and glucagon. The tests for the pancreas are done in order to assess whether or not the pancreas is working.

Lipid testing is common, in particular because the lipid profile can tell a lot about the patient's risk for arteriovascular disease. Lipids store energy as fat and are used to create cell membranes and components of certain vitamins and hormones. The most common lipoproteins found inside the body and detectable in the bloodstream are triglycerides and cholesterol. Some cholesterol is found in the food we eat, while the remainder is made in the liver. There are two types of cholesterol are HDL (high density lipoproteins) and LDL (low density lipoproteins). The purpose of lipid testing is to find the ratio of HDL and LDL as well as to identify the triglyceride level. The findings on a lipid profile can help determine a person's risk for heart disease, stroke, and peripheral vascular disease.

LDL goes out to the cells by means of the bloodstream. Any excess LDL is removed from the bloodstream by HDL and is transported to the liver where it is made into bile acids and removed through the stool. When LDL is too high, plaques form on arterial walls, leading to arterial blockages.

Amylase

Amylase is an enzyme made by the salivary glands and the pancreas. It is usually found in a low quantity in the blood unless there is a blockage or damage to the pancreas or salivary glands. The amylase level is checked whenever there is a suspicion of salivary gland inflammation or pancreatitis/pancreatic cancer. A lipase is checked along with the level of amylase because lipase is only produced by the pancreas and a differentiation of the source of an elevated amylase can be determined. The normal amylase range is between 60 and 180 U/L. Elevated levels of amylase are seen in pancreatic cancer, pancreatitis, mumps, and bowel infarction. It is also found to be elevated in cystic fibrosis, inflamed salivary glands, stomach ulcer, gallstones, ectopic pregnancy, and diabetic ketoacidosis. Low levels of amylase are seen in advanced cystic fibrosis, preeclampsia, and severe liver disease. High levels can be a normal finding in the elderly and in pregnancy. A normal amylase level does not mean there is no pancreatitis.

Lipase

Lipase is produced only in the pancreas and is elevated when the pancreatic duct is blocked or if there is a damaged pancreas. A high level of lipase does not prove the diagnosis of a pancreatic disease and more testing is necessary if the level is elevated. The lipase level can be elevated in pancreatitis, cystic fibrosis, and pancreatic cancer. A normal level of lipase is less than 200 U/L. Lipase can also be elevated in bowel obstructions, gallstones, chronic renal disease, infection, peptic ulcer, cholecystitis, and inflammation.

Cholesterol and Triglycerides

Cholesterol is transported in the blood by means of water soluble lipoproteins. The components checked in a lipid profile include the total cholesterol, LDL cholesterol, HDL cholesterol, very low density lipoprotein (VLDL) and triglycerides. This test is done to determine heart disease risk or the diagnosis of a lipid disorder. Ideally, the blood should be done after fasting for 12 hours.

- Normal cholesterol: less than 240 mg/dL

- Normal HDL: greater than 40 mg/dL

- Normal total cholesterol to HDL ratio is less than 5:1

- Normal LDL: Less than 160 mg/dL

- Normal VLDL: less than 160 mg/dL

- Normal triglycerides: less than 200 mg/dL

Abnormal test findings can be indicative of coronary artery disease, heart attack, lipid disorder or acute coronary syndrome. There are several different genetic lipid disorders that can put one at greater risk for coronary artery disease, stroke and peripheral vascular disease. In addition, elevated triglycerides can be seen in metabolic syndrome.

Chapter 11: Glucose Tests

The pancreatic islet cells produce both insulin and glucagon based on the blood levels of glucose. When glucose levels are high, insulin is produced which puts glucose into the cells and helps glucose into its storage form, glycogen. When glucose levels are low, glucagon is secreted by the pancreas, signaling the liver to break down glycogen into glucose which raises blood sugar levels. Glucagon also results in the cellular release of glucose. In type I diabetes, the islet cells are damaged so the insulin level is low and the glucose level is high. In type II diabetes, the insulin level is high but the glucose level is also high due to cellular resistance to insulin.

C Peptide

C peptide is part of proinsulin and when proinsulin breaks apart, it goes into C peptide and insulin so the level of C peptide is equal to the amount of insulin made by the pancreatic islet cells. The level of C peptide can differentiate between type I and type II diabetes. It can also tell if the patient has an insulinoma or has had successful removal of an insulinoma. The normal C peptide range is between 0.78 and 1.89 ng/mL. High C peptide levels are seen in type II diabetes, Cushing syndrome, or insulinoma. If the C-peptide level is high and the fasting blood glucose is high, the patient has type II diabetes. If the C-peptide is high and the glucose level is low, then the patient should be evaluated for an insulinoma. Low C-peptide levels are seen in Addison's disease, liver disease and type I diabetes. Type II diabetics can develop a low C peptide level over time.

D-xylose Absorption Test

This is a test of absorption of the simple sugar D-xylose from the intestines. It can be checked in a blood or urine sample. If the D-xylose test is positive, an upper GI series is ordered. The test is done by having the patient drink a 25 gram load of D-xylose. Blood is checked for D-xylose after 2 and 5 hours post-ingestion. It is a screening test for malabsorption. The test is done fasting. A normal D-xylose level is 21 to 57 mg/dL. High D-xylose levels are seen in radiation treatment, Hodgkin disease, and scleroderma. Low D-xylose levels are seen in hookworm, malabsorption syndromes, and celiac disease.

Blood Glucose Level

The blood glucose level can vary with many things. When done on a fasting basis, it is a screen for diabetes mellitus. There are four basic glucose tests: 1) Oral glucose tolerance test, which measures glucose levels after a glucose load; 2) Two hour postprandial blood sugar, which measures the blood sugar two hours after eating a meal; 3) Fasting blood sugar done after an 8 hour fast; 4) random blood glucose, which measures blood glucose at any time of the day without regard to meals or food intake. Things that can affect the blood glucose level include illness, activity, smoking, and certain medications, such as prednisone or birth control pills.

A normal fasting blood sugar is 70-99 mg/dL. A normal 2 hour postprandial glucose test is 70-145 mg/dL. A normal random blood sugar test level is 70-125 mg/dL. Diabetes is diagnosed with a fasting blood sugar of 125 mg/dL or greater or 2 hour postprandial glucose level of greater than 199 mg/dL. A random blood glucose level of greater than 199 mg/dL indicates diabetes. Prediabetes is having a fasting blood sugar of between 100 and 125 mg/dL. Fasting blood glucose of less than 40 mg/dL indicates hypoglycemia, an insulinoma, hypothyroidism, Addison disease, malnutrition, cirrhosis, anorexia, or kidney failure.

Glycohemoglobin (HgbA1c)

This test measures the amount of glucose bound to hemoglobin and can be measured at any time. Because the life span of a red blood cell is 120 days, the test is often done only 4 times per year. It can tell if the treatment for diabetes is adequate. It is not a good test for hypoglycemia. A normal hemoglobin A1c level is 4.5 percent to 5.7 percent. Poorly controlled diabetes is indicated by having a glycosylated hemoglobin level of 8 percent or higher.

Chapter 12: Miscellaneous Tests

Serology Testing

This involves testing the blood for antibodies against a foreign substance or to human tissue designated as being foreign, as is seen with autoimmune disease. Serology testing can also tell a person's blood type and if a person has a particular infection.

Immunoglobulins are human antibodies made by lymphocytes in the immune system in response to a foreign antigen, cancer cells, or sensitized human tissue. The immunoglobulin test can measure the amount of IgM and IgG and other immunoglobulins in the bloodstream. Low immunoglobulin levels overall can mean you have an increase in risk of infection.

The five types of immunoglobulins are as follows:
- IgA—found in saliva and tears. It protects the GI tract, the ears, breathing passages, and the eyes. Ten percent of all immunoglobulin is of this type.

- IgD—found in chest and abdominal tissues. Only about 5 percent of all immunoglobulin are of this type.

- IgE—found in skin, mucous membranes, and lungs. It is commonly elevated in people who have allergies. Less than 5 percent of immunoglobulin is of this type.

- IgG—found in all parts of the body. It crosses the placenta and usually indicates a completed recovery from an infection. Eighty percent of all immunoglobulins are of this type.

- IgM—this is found in lymph fluid and blood. It is the immunoglobulin that first responds to an infection. Five percent of all immunoglobulin is of this type.

Immunoglobulin testing is used to detect whether or not a person has or has had an infection, whether or not they have allergies, for autoimmune diseases, multiple myeloma or macroglobulinemia.

Normal levels of IgA are 85-385 mg/dL, IgD less than 8 mg/dL, IgE less than 10-1,421 mcg/dL, IgG between 565-1,765 mg/dL, and IgM between 55 and 375 mg/dL.

Antinuclear Antibody Testing (ANA)

This is a measure of autoimmune diseases. The results will be released a titer. The higher the titer, the greater is the risk that the person has the disease. The normal range is 1:40 or less. High values can mean the incidence of polymyositis, rheumatoid arthritis, lupus, Raynaud's disease, scleroderma, Hashimoto thyroiditis, Vitamin B12 deficiency, Addison disease or hemolytic anemia. Older people and those with a family history of an autoimmune disease may have elevations in the ANA titer.

HIV Testing

HIV infects the CD4+ blood cells, which fight infection. Most HIV is HIV-1 but African cases have HIV-2. HIV is the virus that causes AIDS. The time of exposure to seroconversion can be anywhere from two weeks to six months.

There are many different types of HIV tests, including the ELISA test, which is a screening test for the disease. If the test is negative, the patient does not have HIV. If the test is positive, another ELISA test is performed to rule out a false positive. The Western blot test is a follow up test to see if the positive ELISA test was accurate or not. A polymerase chain reaction or PCR looks for RNA from HIV in the bloodstream. It is the test used to screen blood for infusion (donated blood). The IFA or indirect fluorescent antibody test is done after two positive ELISA tests have been confirmed; it checks for HIV antibodies. There is also a saliva test for HIV present in saliva. These results must always be confirmed by a Western blot test. These tests are done at 6 weeks, three months and six months post-exposure to HIV.

The CD4+ count is used to determine if the immune system has been affected by the HIV virus. A viral load test can also be helpful in determining how much HIV is in the system. These tests together say when the antiretroviral treatment for the HIV infection needs to be started. The normal CD4+ count in unaffected individuals is 600-1,200 cells per microliter. A low CD4+ count means that the immune system is compromised. Antiretroviral treatment is begun when the CD4+ count is less than 200 cells per microliter.

The viral load test checks for the amount of HIV RNA in the patient's blood. There are actually three different types of viral load tests. The first is the branched DNA test; the second is the nucleic acid sequence-based amplification; the third is the reverse-transcriptase polymerase chain reaction. Even with a negative viral load test, the patient can still be infectious.

Rheumatoid Factor

This is an autoantibody test that detects the presence of rheumatoid arthritis. There are two types of RF tests: the nephelometry test and the agglutination test. A person with a positive RF can have no symptoms but is at risk for RA in the future. Symptoms of RA in the absence of a positive RF test should be tested again. Higher RF levels are seen in older adults. The test results are reported as a titer. A normal RF test is 1:40 or less. High levels can also be seen in lupus, malaria, hepatitis, endocarditis, syphilis, vasculitis, mononucleosis, and tuberculosis.

Conclusion

I hope you received a ton of value from this book. Remember, practice makes perfect so you will have to repeat these readings. I am also working on creating some flashcards to send you guys that will help you further with memorizing these lab values! I'm excited to get those out as well.

If you enjoyed this book, would you be kind enough to leave a review on Amazon? Your positive review can help others to see what kinds of helpful resources are out there!

Thank you and good luck on your medical endeavors!

- Chase Hassen

NCLEX: Lab Values

105 Nursing Practice Questions & Rationales to EASILY Crush the NCLEX!

Chase Hassen

Nurse Superhero

© 2015

Disclaimer:

Although the author and publisher have made every effort to ensure that the information in this book was correct at press time, the author and publisher do not assume and hereby disclaim any liability to any party for any loss, damage, or disruption caused by errors or omissions, whether such errors or omissions result from negligence, accident, or any other cause.

This book is not intended as a substitute for the medical advice of physicians. The reader should regularly consult a physician in matters relating to his/her health and particularly with respect to any symptoms that may require diagnosis or medical attention.

Table of Contents

Chapter 1: Lab Values: Questions, Answers, and Rationales

1. You are drawing blood from antecubital vein. In what order do you do these steps?
   a. Clean the puncture sites with alcohol
   b. Remove the tourniquet
   c. Apply the tourniquet to see the veins easier
   d. Insert the needle into the vein with the bevel side up
   e. Apply firm pressure to the site
   f. Attach the appropriate test tube to the needle

Answer: c. a. d f. b. e. First you apply the tourniquet and then you clean the puncture site. Insert the needle into the vein and attach the appropriate test tube to the needle. Remove the tourniquet when the blood has been drawn and apply firm pressure to the site when withdrawing the needle.

2. The client has had their blood drawn and has developed redness and swelling at the injected area. What treatment to you recommend?
   a. Cold packs to the affected area.
   b. Ibuprofen
   c. Tylenol
   d. Warm compresses

Answer: d. The patient has developed phlebitis from the blood draw for which the recommended treatment is warm compresses to the affected area.

Chase Hassen

3. The client needs a blood transfusion and blood typing has not yet been completed. What type of blood do you give the patient?
   a. AB+
   b. O-
   c. O+
   d. B-

Answer: b. O- blood has no antigens on the surface, making it the universal donor kind of blood to give when the actual blood type of the client is not clear.

4. The client has A + blood. What kind of blood can be given to the client in an emergency besides A+ blood?
   a. AB+
   b. AB-
   c. B+
   d. A-

Answer: d. Any blood group that contains a B antigen will not be compatible with the patient's blood. Only A- blood contains antigens that are compatible with A+ blood.

5. The client has had a false positive Rh test. What medication might have caused this?
   a. Levodopa
   b. Amoxicillin
   c. Atropine
   d. Methyl prednisone

Answer: a. Clients on Methyldopa, levodopa or Keflex may have a false positive Rh test.

6. The client is being treated with heparin. What blood test follows the effectiveness of the medication?
   a. Protime
   b. Bleeding time
   c. Partial thromboplastin time
   d. Factor VIII levels

Answer: c. The partial thromboplastin time or PTT is used to evaluate the effectiveness of heparin in thinning the blood.

7. The client is being treated with warfarin. What blood test follows the effectiveness of the medication?
   a. Protime
   b. Bleeding time
   c. Partial thromboplastin time
   d. Factor VIII levels

Answer: a. The protime can be used to measure the effectiveness of warfarin to thin the blood.

8. What partial thromboplastin time indicates that heparin is being effective in thinning the blood?
   a. PTT of 10
   b. PTT of 30
   c. PTT of 40
   d. PTT of 45

Answer: d. A normal PTT is between 30 and 40. A PTT higher than that means that the blood is thin from heparin.

9. A client has a factor deficiency that causes an increased partial thromboplastin time. What factor deficiency exists?
   a. Factor II
   b. Factor V
   c. Factor VII
   d. Factor XII

Answer: c. Factor VII deficiency is associated with a prolonged PTT.

10. A total serum protein level mostly assesses the level of which blood protein?
    a. Beta globulin
    b. Albumin
    c. Alpha globulin
    d. Hemoglobin

Answer: b. Albumin is the most abundant blood protein and is the one that factors most into the total serum protein level.

11. The client is suffering from multiple myeloma. Which blood protein is likely to be elevated?
    a. Globulin
    b. Albumin
    c. Hemoglobin
    d. Estrogen

Answer: a. In multiple myeloma, the serum globulin level will be elevated. The others will not be elevated.

12. The client is said to have a low total protein level if the total protein level is what?
    a. 6.0 g/dL
    b. 4.0 g/dL
    c. 8.0 g/dL
    d. 10.0 g/dL

Answer: b. The normal total serum protein level is 5.5-9.0 g/dL. If the level is 4.0 g/dL it is considered to be too low.

13. The client has low albumin levels. What conditions might be causing this? Select all that apply.
    a. Hypothyroidism
    b. Malnutrition
    c. Kidney disease
    d. Pulmonary edema
    e. Severe burns

Answer: b. c. e. Clients may have low serum albumin levels if they have hyperthyroidism, malnutrition, lupus, kidney disease, liver disease, or severe burns.

14. In assessing a client's blood alcohol level, what is a priority intervention?
    a. Have an officer present for the blood testing.
    b. Do not cleanse the site of blood draw with alcohol.
    c. Compare the blood alcohol level with the breath test.
    d. Ask the client when alcohol was last consumed.

Answer: b. When checking the blood alcohol level, the site of the blood draw should not be swabbed with an alcohol swab.

15. The intoxicated client is unconscious. What is a likely blood alcohol level in this individual?
    a. 0.01
    b. 0.1
    c. 0.2
    d. 0.35

Answer: d. A client with a blood alcohol level of 0.35 is likely to be unconscious.

16. The client has been ordered to have a lead immobilization urine test. What is the purpose of this test?
    a. To check for lead toxicity
    b. To see if chelation therapy is working
    c. To see if lead is being excreted in the urine
    d. To check the blood to urine ratio of lead

Answer: b. The lead immobilization urine test is a test to see if chelation therapy for lead is working.

17. Which things contribute to the serum osmolality?
    a. Hemoglobin
    b. Glucose
    c. Chloride
    d. Sodium
    e. Phosphorus
    f. Magnesium

Answer: b. c. d. The serum glucose, chloride, sodium, protein and bicarbonate levels all contribute to the serum osmolality.

18. The serum osmolality will be low in which of the following conditions?
    a. Dehydration
    b. SIADH
    c. Hypopituitarism
    d. Hypothyroidism

Answer: b. In SIADH (Syndrome of Inappropriate ADH secretion), the kidneys will respond and will cause a lowering of the serum osmolality.

19. The C-reactive protein level has been found to be elevated. What is the next step?
    a. Check a WBC count
    b. Do a serum protein electrophoresis
    c. Do tests to find out the source of the inflammation
    d. Repeat the test in a week

Answer: c. After an elevated C-reactive protein has been identified, the next step is to do further testing to find out the source of the inflammation. The C-reactive protein is not a specific test.

20. The size of the erythrocytes is measured by what lab value?
    a. MCH
    b. MCHC
    c. Hemoglobin
    d. MCV

Answer: d. The size of the erythrocytes is determined by the mean cell volume or MCV.

21. The client has anemia which is microcytic with an increase in RDW. What is the most common cause of this client's condition?
    a. B12 deficiency anemia
    b. Iron deficiency anemia
    c. Folate deficiency anemia
    d. Acute blood loss anemia

Answer: b. The client likely has iron deficiency anemia because the cells are microcytic and the RDW, which is a measure of the different sizes of cells is high, a common finding in iron deficiency.

22. The client has his WBC count measured. In a man, what is a normal WBC count?
    a. 2000-4000 mcL3
    b. 5000-10,000 mcL3
    c. 8000-14,000 mcL3
    d. 10,000-20,000 mcL3

Answer: b. A normal WBC count for a male is 5000-10,000 mcL3

23. The client is having her hematocrit level checked. What is a normal hematocrit for an adult female?
    a. 25-30 percent
    b. 30-40 percent
    c. 37-47 percent
    d. 52-62 percent

Answer: c. The normal hematocrit level for an adult female is 37-47 percent.

24. The female client is having a hemoglobin checked. What is considered an abnormal hemoglobin for an adult female?
    a. 13.0 g/dL
    b. 9.0 g/dL
    c. 12.5 g/dL
    d. 15 g/dL

Answer: b. The normal range for hemoglobin in an adult female is 12-16 g/dL.

25. The client is having a thrombocyte count checked.
    Which values are considered abnormal? Select all that
    apply.
    a. 50,000 mm3
    b. 150,000 mm3
    c. 200,000 mm3
    d. 400,000 mm3
    e. 450,000 mm3
    f. 500,000 mm3

Answer: a. e. f. The normal thrombocyte count for adults and
children is between 150,000 and 400,000 mm3.

26. The client has an elevated WBC count. What might be
    the cause of the elevated count? Select all that apply.
    a. Aplastic anemia
    b. Chemotherapy drugs
    c. Inflammation
    d. Infection
    e. Leukemia
    f. Bone marrow suppression

Answer: c. d. e. Common causes of an elevated WBC count are
inflammation, infection, leukemia, major burns, stress, tissue
damage, and malnutrition.

27. The client has an elevated RBC count. What might be the cause of this condition? Select all that apply.
    a. Alcoholism
    b. Polycythemia vera
    c. Bone marrow suppression
    d. Low altitudes
    e. Smoking
    f. Acute bleeding

Answer: a. b. e. Common causes of an elevated RBC count include alcoholism, polycythemia vera, smoking, dehydration, burns, sweating, vomiting, and carbon monoxide exposure.

28. The clients MCV count is elevated. What might be causes of this? Select all that apply.
    a. Iron deficiency
    b. Acute blood loss
    c. Polycythemia vera
    d. B12 deficiency
    e. Folate deficiency
    f. Anemia of chronic disease

Answer: d. e. Causes of an elevated MCV include B12 and folate deficiency anemias.

29. The client has an elevated B12 level. What might be the cause of this result? Select all that apply.
    a. Pernicious anemia
    b. Fish tapeworm infection
    c. Hepatitis
    d. Cirrhosis
    e. Leukemia
    f. Multiple myeloma

Answer: c. d. e. Hepatitis, cirrhosis, and leukemia can cause elevated B12 levels. The other answers result in low B12 levels.

30. The client is scheduled for a cold agglutinins test. How do you explain the test to the client?
    a. Cold agglutinins testing evaluates the bone marrow function.
    b. Cold agglutinins testing measures antibodies that are active in cold temperatures.
    c. Cold agglutinins testing evaluates the body for inflammation.
    d. Cold agglutinins testing evaluates the platelets ability to clot.

Answer: b. Cold agglutinins testing measures antibodies that are active in cold temperatures. They can result in hemolytic anemia when an individual is exposed to the cold.

31. The client has a low folic acid level. What might be the cause of this low level? Select all that apply.
    a. Alcohol abuse
    b. Macrocytic anemia
    c. Anorexia nervosa
    d. Crohn's disease
    e. Folate supplements
    f. Pregnancy

Answer: a. c. d. Common causes of low folic acid levels include alcohol abuse, anorexia nervosa, Crohn's disease, cirrhosis, celiac disease, kidney disease, and hemolytic anemia.

32. The gastrin test is primarily to evaluate a client for what condition?
    a. Peptic acid disease
    b. Pepsinogen deficiency
    c. Zollinger-Ellison Syndrome
    d. Pepsin deficiency

Answer: c. In Zollinger-Ellison Syndrome, there is a marked elevation in gastrin levels, leading to peptic ulcers.

33. A serum ferritin level is being drawn on a client as a screening test for what condition?
    a. Hemochromatosis
    b. Folate deficiency
    c. B12 deficiency
    d. Polycythemia vera

Answer: a. A serum ferritin level is a screening test for hemochromatosis in which there are elevated iron stores.

34. The client had a Schilling test and the 24 hour urine 12 level was 0. What does this indicate?
    a. The client has inadequate levels of folate.
    b. The client is not absorbing vitamin B12
    c. The client has iron deficiency anemia
    d. This is a normal value for a Schilling test

Answer: b. A 24 hour urine B12 level of 0 in a Schilling test indicates the client is not absorbing vitamin B12 and likely has malabsorption of vitamin B12.

35. The client is suspected of having inflammation. What tests might be done to assess the client for inflammation?
    a. Hematocrit
    b. Lymphocyte count
    c. Erythrocyte sedimentation rate
    d. C reactive protein
    e. WBC
    f. Schilling test

Answer: c. e. e. The erythrocyte sedimentation rate, C reactive protein and WBC can all be indicators of inflammation.

36. Which iron test measures the capacity of blood to carry iron?
    a. Serum iron
    b. TIBC
    c. Ferritin
    d. Transferrin saturation test

Answer: b. The TIBC or total iron binding capacity measures the capacity of blood to carry iron.

37. The client has elevated levels of PTH. What is physiologically occurring? Select all that apply.
    a. Calcium absorption is decreased
    b. Vitamin D is stimulated to increase calcium absorption.
    c. Phosphate levels are increased
    d. Osteoclasts break down bone to increase calcium
    e. Kidneys retain calcium
    f. Calcitonin is stimulated.

Answer: b. d. e. PTH increases calcium by stimulating vitamin D to increase calcium absorption, causing the kidneys to hold onto calcium and causing osteoclasts to break down bone in order to increase calcium. Phosphate levels will decrease as calcium levels rise.

38. The client has a low calcium level. What might be the cause? Select all that apply.
    a. Hyperparathyroidism
    b. Hypoparathyroidism
    c. Osteoporosis
    d. Malabsorption syndrome
    e. Hyperthyroidism
    f. Hypothyroidism

Answer: b. d. Low calcium levels occur in situations of hypoparathyroidism or malabsorption syndrome. Thyroid disease does not affect calcium levels.

NCLEX Takeover

39. The client has had an electrolyte panel. What electrolyte is likely to decrease as calcium increases?
    a. Phosphate
    b. Potassium
    c. Sodium
    d. Chloride

Answer: a. The phosphate level decreases as the calcium level increases.

40. The client is having an electrolyte test that measures calcium. What can affect the results of the test? Select all that apply.
    a. Ingesting milk 8 hours before the test.
    b. Taking vitamin D before the test.
    c. Taking calcium supplements before the test.
    d. Taking a laxative before the test.
    e. Drinking a carbonated beverage before the test.
    f. Exercising before the test.

Answer: a. b. c. Ingesting milk 8 hours before the test, Taking vitamin D before the test and taking calcium supplements before the test can all affect the calcium level when it is measured as part of an electrolyte panel.

41. In explaining what the client should do before having a test for magnesium, what does the nurse say?
    a. Avoid taking laxatives 3 days before the test.
    b. Exercise 2 hours before the test
    c. Don't exercise 2 hours before the test
    d. Avoid eating three days before the test.

Answer: a. When having a magnesium test, the client should avoid taking laxatives 3 days before the test. Exercise does not affect magnesium levels. The test does not have to be done fasting.

42. The nurse should assess to see if the client has taken antibiotics before the test for potassium. Why is this so?
    a. Taking antibiotics mean that the client has a bacterial infection.
    b. Some antibiotics contain potassium.
    c. Patients who take antibiotics have higher than normal levels of potassium.
    d. Patients might vomit during the test.

Answer: b. Some antibiotics contain potassium which might affect the potassium test.

43. The client has an electrolyte panel drawn. Which electrolyte is expected to have an inverse relationship with sodium?
    a. Potassium
    b. Magnesium
    c. Phosphate
    d. Chloride

Answer: a. Potassium has an inverse relationship with sodium.

44. The client is being evaluated for cell lysis syndrome. What electrolyte is used to screen for this condition?
    a. Sodium
    b. Potassium
    c. Magnesium
    d. Phosphate

Answer: b. Potassium is released from the cells during cell lysis syndrome and will be elevated.

45. What is measured in an arterial blood gas measurement? Select all that apply.
    a. Oxygen level
    b. Carbon dioxide level
    c. Bicarbonate level
    d. Potassium level
    e. Sodium level
    f. Magnesium level

Answer: a. b. c. The arterial blood gas measurement measures the oxygen, carbon dioxide, and bicarbonate levels in arterial blood.

46. The client has had an arterial blood gas measurement. What is considered an abnormal blood pH?
    a. 7.30
    b. 7.35
    c. 7.40
    d. 7.45

Answer: a. A normal blood pH is between 7.35 and 7.45. A level of 7.30 is considered too low.

47. What aspect of a blood gas measurement is most active in controlling the blood pH?
    a. Carboxyhemoglobin
    b. Bicarbonate
    c. CO_2
    d. Oxygen

Answer: b. The pH of the blood is determined by the kidney's absorption or excretion of bicarbonate.

48. The client is to have an arterial blood gas measurement. What must the nurse ask of the client before doing the test?
    a. Has the client been taking antibiotics?
    b. Has the client been taking anticoagulants?
    c. Has the client been taking antacid?
    d. Has the client been taking cardiac antiarrhythmics?

Answer: b. Anticoagulant use can greatly increase the amount of time pressure needs to be applied to the arterial puncture site after the test has been drawn.

49. The client is suspected to have carbon monoxide poisoning. What symptoms can be expected? Select all that apply.
    a. Anxiousness
    b. Extreme sleepiness
    c. Headache
    d. Decreased hearing
    e. Confusion
    f. Diarrhea

Answer: b. c. e. Symptoms of CO poisoning include extreme sleepiness, headache, confusion, dizziness, and nausea/vomiting. The other symptoms are not consistent with carbon monoxide poisoning.

50. At what CO level is death imminent?
    a. 20 percent
    b. 30 percent
    c. 50 percent
    d. 60 percent

Answer: d. Death is likely if the carbon monoxide level is at or exceeds 60 percent.

51. What should the nurse tell a client after taking an arterial blood sample? Select all that apply.
    a. You may have a small bruise at the puncture site.
    b. You may feel light headed.
    c. You should not carry heavy objects for 24 hours after the test.
    d. Don't use the affected arm for eating for 8 hours.
    e. The test is being done on the dominant hand.
    f. There is no risk of infection following this test.

Answer: a. b. c. After the arterial blood stick, which ideally should be done on the non-dominant hand, the client may have a small bruise at the puncture site, may feel light headed and should not carry heavy objects for 24 hours following the test. There is a small risk of infection and the client may use the arm for eating after the test.

52. The client has been taking Coumadin at the time of an arterial blood stick. What is the potential result?
    a. Inaccurate test results
    b. The client must take a baby aspirin after the test.
    c. Coagulation times may be longer than ten minutes.
    d. The test should not be performed.

Answer: c. If the client has been taking Coumadin, the coagulation time may be longer than ten minutes so pressure needs to be placed on the site for a longer period of time.

NCLEX Takeover

53. A client is suffering from kidney failure. What test result might be found on the arterial blood gases?
    a. Respiratory alkalosis
    b. Metabolic acidosis
    c. Metabolic alkalosis
    d. Respiratory acidosis

Answer: c. The client is likely to have metabolic alkalosis due to the kidney's lack of excretion of HCO_3-.

54. A client with a CO level of 18 percent will be expected to exhibit what?
    a. Symptoms of carbon monoxide poisoning
    b. No symptoms of carbon monoxide poisoning
    c. Slight symptoms of carbon monoxide poisoning
    d. Severe symptoms of carbon monoxide poisoning.

Answer: b. At a CO level of 18 percent, the client will show no symptoms of carbon monoxide poisoning. Symptoms do not begin to occur until the CO level is in excess of 20 percent.

55. A client has severe diarrhea. What may be found on
    their arterial blood gas evaluation?
    a. Respiratory alkalosis
    b. Metabolic alkalosis
    c. Metabolic acidosis
    d. Respiratory acidosis

Answer: b. Severe diarrhea results in a loss of fluids and a relative
increase in bicarbonate levels.

56. A sign of low bicarbonate levels on an arterial blood
    gas is what?
    a. Low blood pressure
    b. Hyperventilation
    c. Hypoventilation
    d. High blood pressure

Answer: b. The client with a low bicarbonate level has metabolic
acidosis. The lungs respond by hyperventilating in order to blow of
"acidic" CO_2 to keep the pH stable.

57. The client is suspected of having CO poisoning. What test can be done to measure the carboxyhemoglobin level in the blood?
    a. Serum HCO3- level
    b. Carbon monoxide test
    c. Total carbon dioxide test
    d. Arterial blood gases

Answer: b. To evaluate the actual amount of CO in the blood, a carbon monoxide test must be done. ABGs will be inaccurate in the presence of CO and HCO3-/total carbon dioxide testing will not help.

58. The client has a positive Hepatitis A antibody titer. What does this mean?
    a. The client has been exposed to Hepatitis A within the last 7 days.
    b. The client has had the hepatitis A Vaccine a month ago.
    c. The client has active symptoms of hepatitis A.
    d. The client is at risk for hepatitis A viral infection.

Answer: b. The client will have a positive hepatitis A IgM antibody test after exposure to the virus 2 weeks ago or longer or who had the vaccination 2 weeks ago or longer. Symptoms may or may not be present.

59. The client has Hepatitis B testing. Which test indicates that an individual is capable of passing on the hepatitis B virus?
    a. HBsAg
    b. HBsAb IgM
    c. HBsAb IgG
    d. Hepatitis B DNA test

Answer: a. If an individual has a positive HBsAg test, it means they carry the antigen for hepatitis B and can pass the disease along to another through blood exposure or sexual activity. The HBsAb IgM and IgG tests indicate an immunity to the virus. The hepatitis B DNA test is a test to see if the client is responding to hepatitis B treatment.

60. Which blood test is used to screen transfused blood for hepatitis B?
    a. HBsAg
    b. Hepatitis DNA test
    c. HBsAB
    d. HBcAb

Answer: d. The hepatitis B core antibody test (HBcAb) is used to screen blood products for the presence of a hepatitis B infection in the donor blood.

61. The client has an elevated alanine aminotransferase test (ALT). Sources of ALT in the body include what? Select all that apply.
   a. Brain
   b. Heart
   c. Liver
   d. Pancreas
   e. Spleen
   f. Stomach

Answer: b. c. d. Sources of ALT in the body include the liver, heart, pancreas, skeletal muscle, and kidneys.

62. The client has an extremely high level of ALT in the body? What might be the cause?
   a. Barbiturate use
   b. Statin use
   c. Severe liver damage
   d. Exercise before taking the test

Answer: c. Severe liver damage or viral hepatitis can cause extremely high levels of ALT. The other choices will result in mild elevations of the ALT.

63. An 8 year old client has an elevated alkaline phosphatase (ALP) level. What might be the problem?
    a. The client has normal levels of ALP for his age.
    b. The client has a brain tumor.
    c. The client has pancreatitis.
    d. The client has kidney failure.

Answer: a. Children will have elevated ALP levels due to active bone growth. ALP is not found in the brain or pancreas and, while it is found in the kidneys, kidney failure does not result in an elevation of ALP.

64. Very high levels of alkaline phosphatase may be seen in what condition?
    a. Appendicitis
    b. Hepatitis
    c. Lung cancer
    d. Pancreatitis

Answer: b. Very high levels of ALP may be seen in hepatitis, gallstones, obstructive jaundice, liver disease, or cancer metastasized to the liver. It would only be elevated in lung cancer if it has metastasized to the liver. It is not seen in pancreatitis or appendicitis.

65. The client has an elevated ammonia level and a family member asks what this means. How do you respond?
    a. The ammonia level increases after eating.
    b. The ammonia level is increased due to decreased renal excretion of ammonia.
    c. The ammonia level is elevated because the liver cannot turn ammonia into urea.
    d. The ammonia level is because the client is on a low protein diet.

Answer: c. In most cases, an elevated ammonia level means that the liver cannot turn ammonia into urea, which would otherwise be excreted by the kidneys. It is not elevated in a low protein diet and does not increase after eating.

66. The client has an elevated aspartate aminotransferase level (AST). Where is this enzyme found in the body? Select all that apply.
    a. Spleen
    b. Brain
    c. Liver
    d. Heart
    e. GI tract
    f. Muscle tissue

Answer: c. d. f. AST is found in liver, heart, muscle tissue, pancreas, kidneys, and red blood cells.

NCLEX Takeover

67. The client has very high levels of AST. What might be the reason why?
    a. Strenuous exercise before the test
    b. Viral hepatitis
    c. Statin use
    d. Recent IM injection

Answer: b. Very high levels of AST can be seen in liver necrosis and viral hepatitis. The others will cause lesser levels of AST elevation.

68. The client is having a bilirubin test. What is being tested for?
    a. Hemolytic anemia
    b. Cirrhosis
    c. Renal dysfunction
    d. Pancreatitis

Answer: b. The bilirubin level can be evaluated for liver disease, cirrhosis or viral hepatitis.

69. The client is positive for anti-HAV IgM. What does this mean?
    a. The client was recently infected with the hepatitis A virus
    b. The client was infected at some point with the hepatitis A virus
    c. The client was recently infected with the hepatitis B virus
    d. The client was infected at some point with the hepatitis B virus

Answer: a. A positive anti-HAV IgM antibody test indicates a recent infection with hepatitis A. After several weeks, the IgG antibody appears.

70. The client asks what the term "alanine aminotransferase" means in their blood report. You explain that it stands for ALT and is what?
    a. An enzyme found only in the liver
    b. An enzyme found mainly in the liver
    c. A test to determine the amount of carbohydrate stored in the liver
    d. A common test to rule out a recent myocardial infarction

Answer: b. The ALT is an enzyme found mainly in the liver. It can be elevated in an acute myocardial infarction but it is not the primary test used to identify the problem.

Chase Hassen

71. The client has been taking lactulose. What does this mean with regard to an ammonia test?
    a. Lactulose is a laxative that reduces the intestinal bacterial production of ammonia.
    b. Lactulose increases the bacterial production of ammonia in the intestines.
    c. Lactulose interrupts the liver's metabolism of ammonia.
    d. Lactulose binds to ammonia in the bloodstream, reducing the level.

Answer: a. Lactulose is a laxative that reduces the intestinal bacterial production of ammonia so the test won't accurately reflect the liver's input into the ammonia level.

72. The client is having a bilirubin test. What does this test measure?
    a. Only the total bilirubin
    b. The total bilirubin and the direct bilirubin
    c. The total bilirubin and the indirect bilirubin
    d. Only the indirect bilirubin

Answer: b. The bilirubin test measures the total and direct bilirubin. The indirect bilirubin is a calculated value based on the total and direct bilirubin levels.

73. The infant is experiencing physiological jaundice. You tell the parents that this is because:
    a. The newborn is unable to break down red blood cells due to an immaturity of the liver.
    b. The newborn cannot break down red blood cells and needs a blood transfusion.
    c. The newborn has an immature liver and needs a liver transplant.
    d. The mother is infected with hepatitis C.

Answer: a. The newborn is unable to break down red blood cells due to an immaturity of the liver. This resolves in about a week.

74. What does the transcutaneous bilirubin meter measure?
    a. The level of immaturity of the liver.
    b. The presence of liver disease in the newborn.
    c. The level of bilirubin in the newborn.
    d. The amount of direct bilirubin in the blood.

Answer: c. The transcutaneous bilirubin meter is a non-invasive way of detecting the amount of bilirubin in the blood. It measures mostly indirect bilirubin and is usually not a function of liver disease.

75. The ammonia test is being used as a screening tool. The ammonia test can screen for what disease?
    a. Reye's syndrome
    b. Hepatitis A
    c. Hepatitis B
    d. Cirrhosis of the liver

Answer: a. The ammonia test can act as a screening tool for Reye's syndrome. It does not screen for hepatitis and is used in monitoring cirrhosis, not for screening.

76. The client has chest pain and a myocardial infarction is suspected. The best test to detect an ongoing myocardial infarction is what?
    a. The ALT level
    b. The LDH level
    c. An EKG
    d. The serum troponin level

Answer: c. In order to detect an ongoing myocardial infarction, an EKG is warranted. Cardiac enzymes can take hours to show up on a blood test.

77. The client is suspected of suffering from heart failure. A good test to evaluate this client is what?
    a. EKG
    b. CPK
    c. Brain natriuretic peptide (BNP)
    d. Lactate dehydrogenase

Answer: c. The BNP level will be elevated anytime the heart has had to work hard over long periods of time.

78. The client is suspected of having had an acute MI. The CPK is elevated. What is the next logical test to do?
    a. LDH isoenzymes
    b. CPK-MB
    c. ALT
    d. AST

Answer: b. If the CPK level is elevated, it is appropriate to order a CPK-MB test to see if the source of the CPK was the heart or from some other tissue.

79. The client is suspected of having had a myocardial infarction. When are the troponin levels expected to rise?
    a. Within 2 hours
    b. Immediately
    c. Within 6 hours
    d. Within 24 hours

Answer: c. The troponin levels do not rise until 6 hours after the myocardial infarction.

80. The client has an elevated troponin level. What does this indicate?
    a. Skeletal muscle damage
    b. Cardiac muscle injury
    c. Liver cell injury
    d. Chronic heart failure

Answer: b. Troponin is only found in the heart so an elevation is specific to cardiac muscle injury.

81. The client is suspected of having had an MI. When is the CPK-MB level expected to rise?
    a. Immediately
    b. Within 2 hours
    c. Within 6 hours
    d. Within 12 hours

Answer: The CPK-MB level is expected to rise within 2 hours and reduce to normal after 3 days.

82. The healthcare provider has ordered a homocysteine level on a client. You explain to the client that this is a test that assesses:
    a. Whether a client has had an MI recently
    b. If the client is at risk for heart failure
    c. If the client is at risk for pulmonary embolism
    d. If the client is at risk for stroke and myocardial infarction

Answer: d. The homocysteine level measures a client's risk for stroke and myocardial infarction. It does not measure whether or not a client has had a recent MI.

83. The client is scheduled for a renin assay. What is this test for?
   a. To detect the presence of kidney disease.
   b. To identify the cause of hypertension.
   c. To identify the cause of a stroke.
   d. To see if anti-hypertensives are working.

Answer: b. The renin assay can help identify if the kidney's elevated renin level is the cause of hypertension.

84. What must the client do for an accurate renin assay test?
   a. Rest for two hours before the first blood sample is taken and ambulate for two hours before second blood test is taken.
   b. Lay recumbent when the test is taken.
   c. Ambulate for two hours before the first test is taken and rest for two hours before the first test is taken.
   d. Ambulate before both tests are taken.

Answer: a. The client must rest for two hours before the first test is taken and ambulate for two hours before the second blood test is taken. They must be upright when both blood tests are done.

85. Prior to having a homocysteine level assessed, the client needs to:
    a. Be fasting for 12 hours before the test is taken.
    b. Walk ten blocks before the test is administered.
    c. Remain recumbent for 8 hours before the test is taken.
    d. Avoid physical activity before the test is taken.

Answer: a. The client must be fasting for 12 hours before the test is taken. Physical activity plays no role in the test results.

86. What enzymes are mostly found in cardiac muscle?
    a. Troponin and CPK-MB
    b. CPK and creatine phosphokinase
    c. Troponin and LDH
    d. AST and ALT

Answer: a. The two enzymes primarily found in cardiac muscle are troponin and CPK-MB.

87. Why would recent surgery have a negative effect on cardiac enzyme studies?
    a. The client must be NPO when the blood sample is taken.
    b. Surgery adds stress to the cardiac muscle.
    c. Surgery disrupts skeletal muscle, which releases enzymes in muscle tissue.
    d. Surgery weakens the client's immune system.

Answer: c. Surgery disrupts skeletal muscle which contains some of the same enzymes as cardiac muscle.

88. IgA antibodies are found where in the body?
    a. Tears, digestive tract and saliva
    b. Spleen
    c. Liver
    d. Red blood cells

Answer: a. IgA antibodies are found in tears, the digestive tract, the vagina, and saliva. They protect these areas from foreign invaders.

89. The client has an elevated IgE antibody titer. Which antibody type is mostly associated with allergens?
    a. IgA
    b. IgG
    c. IgE
    d. IgD

Answer: c. IgE antibodies are mainly associated with allergens and allergies, as well as parasitic infections.

90. The client has a positive IgM antibody titer but a negative IgG antibody titer. What is the IgM antibody titer most associated with?
    a. Longstanding immunity against an infectious disease.
    b. A first response antibody to an infection.
    c. The client is not immune to the infection.
    d. The client is susceptible to getting the infection.

Answer: b. The IgM antibody is the first antibody response to an infection. IgG antibodies indicate a longstanding immunity against an infectious disease.

91. Immunoglobulins are screening tests for what diseases? Select all that apply.
    a. Acute myocardial infarction.
    b. Bone marrow cancer.
    c. Autoimmune diseases
    d. Allergies
    e. Multiple myeloma
    f. Type II diabetes

Answer: c. d. e. Immunoglobulin testing involves screening for autoimmune diseases, allergies, multiple myeloma and macroglobulinemia.

92. Elevated IgE levels can indicate what conditions? Select all that apply.
    a. Multiple myeloma
    b. Rheumatoid arthritis
    c. Asthma
    d. Parasitic infections
    e. Cirrhosis
    f. Allergic reaction

Answer: c. d. f. Elevated IgE antibodies can be seen in asthma, parasitic infections, and allergic reactions.

93. Elevated IgD antibody levels can indicate what disease?
    a. Rheumatoid arthritis
    b. Asthma
    c. Chronic hepatitis
    d. Multiple myeloma

Answer: d. Elevated IgD antibody levels can be seen in multiple myeloma.

94. The physician will order an antinuclear antibody titer in a client suspected of having what?
    a. Type II diabetes
    b. Systemic lupus erythematosus
    c. Hypothyroidism
    d. Irritable bowel syndrome

Answer: b. An elevated antinuclear antibody titer can be seen in autoimmune diseases such as systemic lupus erythematosus or SLE.

95. The client has an ANA titer of 1:40. What does a titer indicate?
    a. A titer specifies how much of a sample of blood is diluted before the antibodies are no longer detected.
    b. A titer indicates the absolute value of an antibody in the blood.
    c. A titer is low when the client has the disease.
    d. A titer is a comparison of the client's blood with a control sample.

Answer: a. A titer specifies how much of a sample of blood is diluted before the antibodies are no longer detected. The higher the titer, the greater is the chance the client has the disease.

96. The client has been exposed to HIV. The seroconversion period between the time the client is exposed and the client shows seropositivity is what?
    a. 1-2 days
    b. 1-2 weeks
    c. 2 weeks to 6 months
    d. 6 months to a year

Answer: c. The seroconversion period for HIV is 2 weeks to 6 months during which the client can pass on the disease to another.

97. The client is being screened for HIV. The first test used to screen for HIV is what test?
    a. The HIV RNA test
    b. The Western Blot analysis
    c. The polymerase chain reaction test
    d. The enzyme-linked immunosorbent test (ELISA)

Answer: d. The ELISA test is the first screening test used to identify HIV. It is backed up by the Western Blot test. The HIV RNA test evaluates the viral load.

98. Which test is used to screen blood and organ products for HIV?
    a. The polymerase chain reaction
    b. The ELISA
    c. The Western blot test
    d. The HIV RNA test

Answer: a. The polymerase chain reaction is used to identify a recent HIV infection and is the test used to screen blood and organ products for HIV.

99. The client has been diagnosed with HIV. What test is done to see how severely the HIV infection is progressing?
    a. CD4+ count
    b. ELISA
    c. Western blot test
    d. Polymerase chain reaction test

Answer: a. The CD4+ count can tell how severe an HIV infection is. A viral load level can do the same thing. The other tests are screening tests for HIV.

100. What is true of a positive ELISA test for HIV?
    a. A positive ELISA test means the client is HIV positive.
    b. A positive ELISA test is followed by a polymerase chain reaction test.
    c. A positive ELISA test is repeated and if still positive, a Western blot test is performed.
    d. A positive ELISA test means that the client has AIDS.

Answer: c. A positive ELISA test must be repeated. If it is still positive, a Western blot test is performed to make the identification of an HIV positive client.

101.   What is the purpose of checking the CD4+ count in an HIV positive client?
   a. To see if the client has an opportunistic infection.
   b. To determine when to start antiretroviral treatment.
   c. To see if the PCR test was accurate.
   d. To see what the client's viral load is.

Answer: b. The CD4+ count is assessed in a client to see when to start antiretroviral treatment.

102.   The client is having a rheumatoid factor checked. What is the purpose of this test?
   a. To see if the client has lupus.
   b. To see if the client has been effectively treated with anti-rheumatoid arthritis drugs.
   c. To determine if the person's arthritis is from rheumatoid arthritis.
   d. To recheck the antinuclear antibody test.

Answer: c. The purpose of the rheumatoid factor is to see if the client's arthritis is from rheumatoid arthritis. Once it is positive, it will always remain positive.

103.   The client is having an ANA titer done. What does this measure?
   a. Antibodies that destroy bacteria
   b. Antibodies that destroy viruses
   c. Antibodies that destroy the body's own cells
   d. Antibodies that destroy allergens

Answer: c. The ANA titer measures antibodies that destroy the body's own cells.

104.   Why is the viral load measurement for HIV performed?
   a. To confirm the diagnosis of AIDS
   b. To confirm a positive ELISA test
   c. To determine if the HIV RNA levels are increasing, stabilized or decreasing
   d. To determine a client's ability to pass on the HIV infection.

Answer: c. The viral load measurement determines if the HIV RNA levels are increasing, stabilized or decreasing. It does not tell if a person can pass on the HIV infection and does not confirm a positive ELISA test.

105.   What happens when a client has hypothalamic dysfunction and no longer produces corticotropin-releasing hormone?
a. The levels of epinephrine and norepinephrine go down.
b. The cortisol level increases.
c. The stimulation of the pituitary gland is increased.
d. ACTH levels fall.

Answer: d. When CRH is no longer produced, ACTH is not triggered to be released by the pituitary gland and cortisol levels fall.

Congrats! You did it! Remember, practice makes perfect so you may want to repeat these questions to make you feel more confident for the big exam day. If you enjoyed this book, would you be kind enough to leave a review on Amazon? Your positive review can help others to see what kinds of helpful resources are out there!

Fluid and Electrolytes

24 Hours or Less to Absolutely Crush the NCLEX Exam!

Chase Hassen

Nurse Superhero

© 2015

Disclaimer:

Although the author and publisher have made every effort to ensure that the information in this book was correct at press time, the author and publisher do not assume and hereby disclaim any liability to any party for any loss, damage, or disruption caused by errors or omissions, whether such errors or omissions result from negligence, accident, or any other cause.

This book is not intended as a substitute for the medical advice of physicians. The reader should regularly consult a physician in matters relating to his/her health and particularly with respect to any symptoms that may require diagnosis or medical attention.

NCLEX®, NCLEX®-RN, and NCLEX®-PN are registered trademarks of the National Council of State Boards of Nursing, Inc. They hold no affiliation with this product.

Table of Contents

CHAPTER 5:

CHLORIDE

19. WHAT DOES CHLORIDE DO IN THE BODY?
20. LOW CHLORIDE LEVELS
21. HIGH CHLORIDE LEVELS
22. WHERE DO WE GET CHLORIDE?
23. TESTING FOR CHLORIDE IN THE BLOOD AND URINE
24. NORMAL VALUES OF CHLORIDE IN THE BODY

CHAPTER 6:

POTASSIUM

25. USES OF POTASSIUM IN THE BODY
26. CAUSES OF HYPOKALEMIA
27. SYMPTOMS OF HYPOKALEMIA
28. TREATMENT OF HYPOKALEMIA
29. PREVENTING LOW POTASSIUM CONDITIONS
30. HYPERKALEMIA
31. SYMPTOMS OF HYPERKALEMIA
32. TREATMENT OF HIGH POTASSIUM LEVELS
33. BENEFITS OF POTASSIUM
34. TAKING POTASSIUM SUPPLEMENTS

CHAPTER 7:

MAGNESIUM

35. MAGNESIUM SOURCES
36. LOW MAGNESIUM LEVELS
37. HIGH MAGNESIUM LEVELS
38. MEDICATION INTERACTIONS
39. DIETARY INTAKE OF MAGNESIUM

CHAPTER 8:

CALCIUM

40. PURPOSES OF CALCIUM IN THE BODY

CHAPTER 9:

PHOSPHORUS

CHAPTER 10:

CONCLUSION

Chapter 1:
Introduction

Fluid and electrolyte balance is a very important part of what the body needs to do in order to stay healthy. Fluid is a necessary part of every organ and cell, and fluid makes up much of the extracellular milieu, especially in the blood stream and interstitial fluid (the fluid outside of the cells but not in the bloodstream). Electrolytes represent the mineral content of the bodily fluid. The minerals are in their ionized form, meaning they are represented as mineral ions with an electric charge that makes the mineral part of a salt, acid or base within the body.

For example, sodium and chloride are charged as being positive and negative, respectively. They therefore have a great affinity for one another. When sodium levels are high, for example, there will be a corresponding elevation in chloride. Potassium and chloride are commonly found together within the cells but not so much outside of the cells.

To make matters interesting, there is a great difference in the concentration of electrolytes when comparing the content of electrolytes in the cells as opposed to out of the cells. This difference is maintained by tiny pumps which constantly and instantaneously react to changes in electrolytes within the cells, pumping in potassium and pumping out sodium and their corresponding negatively charged ion. Water balance within the cells is balanced purely by passive movement across the cell membrane.

Which mineral ions are where in the body? The main intracellular ions (charged electrolytes) include potassium, magnesium, phosphorus and sulfate, represented as $K+$, Mg^{2+}, HPO^{2-} and SO_4-, respectively. On the other hand, extracellular ions are primarily sodium, calcium, magnesium, chloride and bicarbonate, represented as Na+, Ca²⁺, Mg²⁺, Cl- and HCO3-, respectively. These ions not only are attracted to each other (positive ions are attracted to negative ions) but they are attracted to any charged molecule in the system, making for electrochemically neutral environment both inside and outside the cells.

Besides their function as salts in the body, electrolytes can also make up parts of the acids and bases within the cells and body tissues. Acid-base neutrality with a pH of about 7.4 is necessary within the body for the proper environment for cellular and extracellular enzymatic processes so that, if the electrolytes are not at their proper concentration and the pH level fails to remain at optimal, the enzymatic activity of various body enzymes can be severely compromised.

Humans, as well as nearly all animal forms, require that even subtle changes in electrolytes must be adjusted so as to keep the proper amounts of the various electrolyte salts within the body. These adjustments are particularly important for proper muscle function and nerve function.

Muscle function and the nerves of the body depend on a specific body pH in order to function. This pH balance is maintained by the salts (electrolyte salts) of the body. If the pH is too low or too high, these bodily functions don't work properly. For an example, consider muscle contractions. In order for muscles to contract properly, there must be sufficient amounts of calcium ions, potassium ions and sodium ions. If these are not in their proper concentration, one can develop muscle weakness or an excess of muscle contraction (tetany). Situations of electrolyte imbalance can be life threatening. For this reason, electrolyte imbalances are treated using oral or IV methods.

If a person suffers from an electrolyte imbalance, it can mean that some part of the body's regulating mechanism in maintaining the proper levels of electrolytes is not working properly. Hormones that regulate electrolyte balance include antidiuretic hormone, parathyroid hormone, and aldosterone. In this book, we will discuss these regulating hormones and what happens when they are insufficient or found in excess quantities.

In order for electrolytes to be in the proper concentrations in the body, one must neither be over hydrated nor dehydrated. The kidneys are mostly responsible for keeping the body hydrated to a proper degree. In situations of dehydration or over hydration, the concentrations of the various salts are affected and there can be serious neurological complications, muscle disturbances and heart problems. These situations often call for immediate medical emergency treatment in order to restore the proper electrolyte and water balance.

9.Measuring Electrolyte Levels

For all of the available electrolytes, there are blood tests available to check their level. In fact, part of a basic chemistry profile is the measurements of the various electrolytes of the body. This is done using ion-selective electrode technology that can tell the difference between the different electrically-charged ions. Along with the electrolyte content checked on a blood test, the kidney function is also assessed as the kidneys are partly responsible for what the electrolyte concentration is.

Normally, just the sodium and potassium levels are evaluated with the chloride level calculated from the sodium level provided by the machine. An exception to this is when doing arterial blood gases, in which the chloride level is measured directly along with the blood gas interpretation.

A urine test can also be assessed to see if the electrolytes are properly balanced. When a specific gravity test is done on a urine sample, it can tell if there is an electrolyte imbalance occurring.

When Rehydration is Necessary

In situations of low water content of the body, this usually occurs along with a loss of sodium and potassium, which are excreted in sweat and by the kidneys. If IV supplementation is necessary, it is usually done by hanging a bag of normal saline (which has the proper amount of sodium chloride in the solution and infusing it directly into a peripheral vein. Often potassium is added to the bag of normal saline to make a balanced salt solution for the bloodstream.

Rehydration can also be done orally, if the individual can take in fluids. Water containing sugar for fuel and electrolytes such as is found in oral rehydration solutions like PowerAde and Gatorade can help rehydrate the individual quickly and effectively. Electrolytes can also be given in the form of coconut water, nuts, milk, and fruit juices. Many vegetables and fruits contain electrolytes, whether they be taken whole placed in a juicer. Along with the electrolyte- containing foods, you should drink plenty of water in order to add water to the system.

Dehydration appropriate for oral intake can be a result of exercising too much, sweating in the heat, or even drinking too much alcohol, which acts as a diuretic, resulting in a negative water balance. Each of these conditions lends itself to oral rehydration as long as the individual is conscious and has normal swallowing reflexes.

In this book, we will look at the various electrolytes in the body and find out how they are regulated. We will look at what happens when the different electrolytes are out of balance and will study the purposes of the different electrolytes.

Chapter 2:
Water Balance in the Body

Our body contains more water in it than you might expect. It is estimated that more than half of all our weight is strictly in the form of water. Women have a lesser water percentage than men (55 percent when compared to men at 60 percent. This is because women have more fat in proportion to other body tissues and because fat cells have a lesser percentage of water in them when compared to other types of cells. Children contain more water by percentage at 70 percent when compared to adults; older adults have a lower percentage of body water than younger adults. On average, a 150 pound male has about 10 gallons of water in his system, of which 2/3 to 3/4 is in the cells, with the rest as part of the interstitial fluid (at 7 gallons) or as blood (about one gallon). Water can shift rapidly from one fluid space to another through the process of osmosis.

Because our kidneys constantly excrete water, we must make up for the losses by drinking water in any form. Without proper water intake, the kidneys eventually shut down, we get dehydrated, and we run the risk of electrolyte disturbances that can cause further disarray when it comes to bodily functions. It is better to drink too much water than to drink too little; our kidneys get rid of excess water quite readily as long as they are functioning properly.

Gains and Losses of Water

Water is taken in primarily by drinking water-containing foods. The water is absorbed from the gastrointestinal tract into the bloodstream, where it is distributed where it is needed. Much smaller amounts of water are byproducts of cellular metabolism. This amount of water usually remains in the cell in which the metabolism occurred.

Water is lost by the body in several different ways. The primary way we lose water is through the kidneys, which can filter and excrete many gallons of water in the urine each day, if necessary. Water is also lost through skin evaporation—about 1.5 pints per day. More is lost if we are sweating in the heat. Water is also more humidified going out of the lungs when compared to water taken in through the air, so we lose a small amount of water just in the act of breathing.

Some water is lost through the stool but this varies from person to person. Severe diarrhea can actually result in dehydration as there is not a normal mechanism to conserve water in the GI tract when an inflammatory process in the gut results in water rushing through the GI tract from the blood and into the stool. Vomiting excessively can lead to dehydration as well as diarrhea. Dehydration requires oral or IV water replacement, preferably before the dehydration becomes too severe. If the dehydration comes in the form of excessive vomiting, fluids must be given by IV so that they stay in the system.

Signs and Symptoms of Dehydration

If you become dehydrated for whatever reason, these are the signs and symptoms you might expect to have:

- An increase in thirst
- Feeling sleepy or tired
- Having a dry mouth
- Feeling dizzy
- Having a low urine output with dark yellow urine
- Having no tears when crying
- Having a headache
- Having extremely dry skin with increased "tenting" of the skin when the skin of the back of the hand is pinched

- If you are impaired as to your level of consciousness, you may not feel thirsty and this can impact your ability to take in enough water; instead, IV hydration may be necessary.

- Severe dehydration has additional symptoms than those listed above. A severely dehydrated patient may have:

  · A severe lack of urine output of deeply-colored urine

  · Rapid heart rate

  · A drop in blood pressure when standing (also called orthostatic hypotension)

  · Dizziness that is worse upon standing

  · Confusion, lethargy or coma

  · Fever

  · Low skin elasticity

  · Seizures

  · Shock

These symptoms require immediate IV hydration so as to save the person from dying of their dehydration.

10. Electrolytes in the Body Water

The water in the body has many different substances in it, particularly electrolytes in the form of sodium salts. There is a strong connection between the balance of water and the balance of electrolytes in the body. Because the electrolyte balance is a greater priority, the body will adjust itself as much as is possible to keep the electrolyte concentration the same. If for example, you have an elevation in sodium in the bloodstream, you will experience a desire to drink water in order to dilute out the over-saturated blood stream. The kidneys will also hold onto water so the sodium concentration can be improved.

There is a brain hormone located in the pituitary gland known as vasopressin or antidiuretic hormone (ADH) that is secreted whenever the body senses it is dehydrated. The elevated ADH level will trigger the kidneys to hold onto more water. As you become more hydrated ADH levels fall back down. On the other hand, if the sodium content of the blood is too low, the kidneys are signaled by low levels of ADH to excrete additional water so that the sodium electrolyte balance is restored.

11.Balancing Water in the System

Water is one of the few body molecules that moves passively through osmosis to all areas and compartments of the body. This means that if a cell or body tissue is low in water, the gradient of water is off and water will naturally flow from one area of the body to the needed area. Because the sodium and other electrolyte content of the bloodstream needs to be controlled above all things, there is a natural tendency for blood to passively flow from the cells and interstitial tissue into the bloodstream to maintain normal electrolyte levels.

Chapter 3:
Introduction to Electrolytes

As mentioned, electrolytes are mineral salts that are ionized to form salt, acids and bases in the body. Electrolytes are important in creating the optimum acid-base balance in the body so that enzymes, which have a narrow acceptable pH range, get a chance to continue doing their job. It also means that electrolytes help control the flow of fluid into and out of the cells and various body tissues. When you become dehydrated, for example, it is the elevation in sodium content in the bloodstream that triggers the pituitary gland to secrete more ADH to decrease urine output by the kidneys.

Electrolytes are charged particles of minerals not usually found in their natural non-ionized state in real life. As ions (charged particles), electrolytes have a natural affinity for oppositely charged particles in the system. Sodium can connect with chloride or bicarbonate in the body, depending on need. Electrolytes do not naturally occur ionized without some sort of matching, oppositely charged electrolyte attached to it.

Electrolytes play an important role in cellular metabolism and help the cells maintain cell membrane stability. The body would not function at all without electrolytes, which are found in every fluid space in the body. Sodium chloride is the most common electrolyte salt outside of the cells, whereas potassium chloride is the most common electrolyte within cells. Your body needs this gradient of electrolytes in order to help muscles contract and to help nerve cells generate the electrochemical "current" required to pass impulses from one nerve cell to another. Almost all cellular and extracellular activities in the body are dependent on a certain concentration of salts (electrolytes).

As mentioned, the concentration of sodium, potassium and chloride in the bloodstream need to be critically managed. There are sensors within the kidneys that secrete the hormone renin that helps to keep the electrolyte content of the body within normal limits. Other important hormones in the management of electrolyte content are aldosterone (secreted by the adrenal gland), angiotensin (secreted by the brain, lung and heart tissues), and ADH (secreted by the pituitary gland).

12.The Renin-Angiotensin System

This is a system that operates in order to restore blood pressure when it drops due to any reason, including dehydration or sudden blood loss. When the blood pressure drops, cells in the kidneys secrete the hormone renin in order to restore blood pressure to normal values. Renin attaches to angiotensinogen (which is a hormone secreted by the liver) to form a molecule called angiotensin

- This increases the blood pressure of the system by constricting blood vessels, allowing for an increase in blood pressure. There are medications available for people who have high blood pressure called ACE inhibitors or angiotensin-converting enzyme inhibitors. They block the formation of another molecule called angiotensin II which is the end-point of this system. There are also angiotensin II inhibitors made by pharmaceutical companies that also help to reduce blood pressure by blocking the direct activity of angiotensin II on the blood vessels. Angiotensin-converting enzyme (ACE) is secreted by the lungs.

13.The Function of Aldosterone

Aldosterone is also secreted by the adrenal glands when the person's blood pressure is too low. It causes the kidneys to secrete less water, also raising the blood pressure. It also regulates sodium reuptake in the kidneys so that, if sodium is low, it can decrease the amount of sodium lost by the kidneys and can increase sodium levels in the body. Indirectly it also regulates the hydrogen and potassium levels in the body, effectively regulating the blood pH.

Chapter 4:
Sodium

Sodium is a mineral salt found in high concentrations in the bloodstream and in the interstitial fluid. It is used to keep water in these areas through osmosis and is important in the functioning of the muscles and nerves of the body.

About 85 percent of all body sodium is found in the lymph fluid and blood. Lesser concentrations of sodium are found within the cells. The levels of sodium in the bloodstream are tightly controlled by a aldosterone, a hormone secreted by the adrenal glands. When the sodium level gets low, aldosterone send a signal to the kidneys that tell it to conserve sodium so it isn't lost in the urine. Another source of sodium loss is through sweating; however, this is not controlled and is not a large amount of loss when compared to the kidneys.

We get sodium through our food as sodium in the form of sodium chloride is added to a lot of cooked and premade foods you eat. You can also get sodium in the form of sodium bicarbonate, which is commonly known as baking soda. Medications contain sodium in them, such as toothpaste, mouthwash, laxatives and aspirin.

Sodium in the bloodstream is often paired with chloride to make the common salt, sodium chloride; however, it can be paired with any positively charged molecule including bicarbonate. Because sodium levels need to be tightly regulated, routine blood tests often contain a test for the amount of sodium and chloride in the blood.

A simple, non-fasting blood test can be done in order to determine the level of sodium in the bloodstream. The normal sodium level is about 135-145 mEq/ l, although the actual normal range can vary from testing instrument to testing instrument. When getting your sodium level, check the reference range listed along with your value.

14.Hypernatremia

Hypernatremia is the medical term for high sodium levels. Usually this is not caused by having too much sodium in the body but rather from a loss of water in the body. The main cause of hypernatremia is dehydration where more water than salt is lost from the body so that the relative concentration of sodium is higher than normal.

You can lose water through sweating, diarrhea, urine, and through the expiration of humidified air from the lungs. You can also rarely get hypernatremia through an excessive intake of salt such as when you consume sea water or large amounts of sodium in the diet. For example, eating a lot of soy sauce can contribute to getting too much sodium in the body. This is uncommon, however.

When you experience a rise in sodium concentration in the bloodstream, it triggers the thirst response and you will feel an inordinate need to take in free water. The addition of free water from the gastrointestinal tract will allow for a lowering of the sodium content to normal levels. Hypernatremia is more common in infants, the elderly and those who lack the mental status to drink water or to recognize the need to drink water. Infants and those who suffer from a mental impairment such as Alzheimer's disease generally lack an intact mechanism to recognize that thirst has occurred or cannot get water into their bodies on their own.

15.Signs and Symptoms of Hypernatremia

High sodium levels can cause symptoms, some of which are not very obvious. When you suffer from hypernatremia, you can experience the following symptoms:

6. Weakness

7. Irritability

8. Lethargy

9. Swelling of the tissues

10.   Excitability of the nerves and muscles

11.   Seizures

12.   Coma, often referred to as a hyperosmolar coma

Symptoms can occur with mild elevations of the sodium level, with severe symptoms occurring when the level of sodium reaches 155 mEq/L or more. When the sodium level reaches 180 mEq/ L or greater, the mortality rate is generally quite high, not necessarily from the absolute value of the sodium concentration but because of the underlying and coexisting conditions related to having high sodium concentrations.

16. Causes of Hypernatremia

You can get hypernatremia from a variety of medical causes, including:

- Low intake of enough water to balance the sodium concentration. This is more common in the disabled or elderly population who cannot get free water for themselves due to their disability or to a loss of the thirst response.

- A loss of sodium in the urine that commonly is associated with elevated glucose concentrations. The kidneys must get rid of the glucose and water must go along with that. Sodium stays behind, resulting in a higher concentration of sodium in the bloodstream.

- Extreme sweating results in more water loss than sodium, so you end up with a higher concentration of sodium in the bloodstream.

- Extreme levels of diarrhea which results in more water loss than sodium. The sodium level will be higher in this situation.

- Diabetes insipidus. This is a condition where the body makes little vasopressin in the pituitary gland or when the kidneys do not normally respond to the vasopressin secreted by the pituitary gland.

- Intake of hyperosmolar water. This can be caused when a person takes on too much seawater or receives too much sodium bicarbonate while being resuscitated from a cardiovascular arrest. Seawater contains more sodium in it than the human body so it should not be consumed, even if you are thirsty.

- Salt poisoning. Sometimes young children ingest too much salt so that they will become hypernatremic.

- A rare condition called Conn's syndrome. These people have too much aldosterone in their system and, when faced with a restriction of free water, tend to become hypernatremic.

- Diuretics tend to cause a relatively greater loss of water when compared to sodium so sodium levels increase in the bloodstream.

17.Treatment of Hypernatremia

When a person develops hypernatremia, the treatment of choice is oral or IV free water. Rarely is this given just as free water (when given by IV) but must be given in the form of a dilute solution of dextrose sugar or half normal saline. It is important not to rapidly correct the state of hypernatremia because this can result in rapid shifts of sodium and water within the cells and interstitial fluid so the sodium level must be slowly returned to normal. Water can flow into brain cells when the hypernatremia is fixed too fast, resulting in swelling of the brain and the chance of getting seizures or permanent damage to the brain. The correction of hypernatremia must be done slowly with frequent sodium concentration measurements as the process is happening.

18.Causes of Hyponatremia (Low Sodium)

Low sodium values occur because of excessive sweating, in which you lose sodium as part of salty sweat. If you have severe burns, these will cause fluid loss through the burned skin; an excess of sodium can be lost when compared to water so the sodium levels become low. Poor nutrition is a more rare cause of hyponatremia. There is a medical/psychiatric illness called polydipsia, in which a person drinks excessive amounts of water, diluting out the blood and interstitial fluid.

More uncommon causes of hyponatremia include the following underlying diseases:

· Adrenal failure

· Thyroid gland dysfunction (low thyroid conditions)

· Kidney failure

· Cystic fibrosis

· Liver cirrhosis

· SIADH, which is a syndrome of inappropriate secretion of the hormone, ADH

The treatment of low sodium is to gradually replace the sodium intake, orally or by IV. Like hypernatremia, the treatment of hyponatremia by IV needs to be done slowly so that the sodium and fluid shifts don't adversely affect the cells of the body, particularly the brain.

Sudden changes in sodium level result in more severe and noticeable symptoms when compared to changing sodium levels gradually. Sudden changes in sodium level can result in poor energy levels, confusion, seizures or death.

In order to find out if the kidneys are participating in having too much sodium or too little sodium in the bloodstream, a test is done of the creatinine level of the blood and the urine. These two levels are compared. If there is sodium being excreted in the urine in amounts not appropriate for either low or high sodium in the bloodstream, kidney failure needs to be considered as part of the reason the person has abnormal sodium levels.

Chapter 5:
Chloride

Chloride is the main negative ion in the body, both in the cells and out of the cells. The rise and fall of chloride closely mimics the rise and fall of sodium as they often are found together in an ionic bond within the body tissues. Chloride, in fact, makes up about 70 percent of the normal body negative ions. Chloride makes up about 0.15 percent of the human total body weight, or about 115 grams of chloride. Every day, we take in close to 900 milligrams of chloride per day.

Chloride is one of the major electrolyte ions in the body, found in all areas of the body, paired with either sodium (outside of the cells) or potassium (within the cells). Chloride is responsible, along with the positive ions Na+ and K+, for the electrical messaging between cells, primarily the muscle cells and nerve cells.

19. What does chloride do in the body?

Chloride helps maintain proper osmolality in the body. It also combines with the hydrogen iron in order to make hydrochloric acid, which is a major factor in digestion in the stomach. Hydrochloric acid breaks down ingested proteins, activates intrinsic factor in the stomach, responsible for the body's uptake of vitamin B12. It is transported via chloride channels in the stomach in exchange for bicarbonate, which is another negatively charged ion, in order to create the gradient between hydrochloric acid and sodium hydrochloride outside of the stomach.

Chloride also helps to maintain the pH balance of the bloodstream by actively and passively passing through the red blood cells in exchange for hydrochloride ions so that the body can maintain a pH balance in the bloodstream of around 7.4. In addition, it aids in the release of CO_2 in the respiratory system and helps support the electrical activity that allows for messages to travel from one nerve cell to another or from one muscle cell to another muscle cell. You can't have an excess of ions, positive or negative, in the body, so chloride acts as the primary mineral element within the interstitial fluids, cellular fluids, and the bloodstream.

20. Low Chloride Levels

It is rare to have a chloride deficiency in the body and, when it is low, it usually goes along with a deficiency of sodium as well. Low chloride levels can lead to alkalization of the bloodstream, in which the pH rises above 7.4. This can be life threatening because many enzymes and bodily processes are very dependent upon the pH of the environment and when they don't function well, the body suffers. A common cause of alkalosis of the bloodstream is when one has excessive sodium and chloride ions lost as sodium chloride in the sweat or whenever there is extensive fluid volume loss during prolonged diarrhea and/or vomiting.

Decreased causes of low chloride concentration include:

10. Addison's disease

11. SIADH (syndrome of inappropriate ADH secretion)

12. Metabolic alkalosis

13. Persistent vomiting

14. Congestive heart failure

Symptoms of hypochloremia or low chloride content in the body include irritability leading to lethargy, loss of appetite and dehydration. You can get hypochloremia in much the same way as losses of sodium are incurred—mainly through serious burn injuries, diseases of water overload and starvation, with wasting of the body tissues. Infants can develop hypochloremia if they drink formula that does not contain enough chloride in it. This can cause the infant to fail to thrive, have weakness and exhibit anorexia.

21.High Chloride Levels

It is possible to have high chloride levels in the body, especially when one consumes large amounts of either sodium chloride (table salt) or potassium chloride (salt substitute). Signs and symptoms of an elevated chloride level include high blood pressure and edema (fluid retention). Fortunately, this is a rare condition as the kidneys are usually able to excrete any excess chloride along with sodium or potassium in the form of NaCl or KCl. Another cause of chloride toxicity is congestive heart failure, which can be from disordered metabolism of sodium chloride. Certain kidney diseases hang on to too much chloride, causing hyperchloremia. Most people do not develop a very high level of chloride because their kidneys can excrete any excess chloride in the system, balancing the sodium levels at the same time

Common causes of high chloride in the body include:

11. Excessive salt intake

12. Renal disease

13. Dehydration (such as is seen in vomiting and diarrhea

14. Hyperparathyroidism (an overactive parathyroid gland)

22.Where do we get chloride?

Chloride is found as a part of sodium chloride or table salt. Whenever we consume salty foods, we are causing a relative increase in both sodium and chloride in the blood and interstitial fluids. If you take a salt substitute, such as potassium chloride, you get a matching rise in both potassium and chloride. In this form, the potassium chloride or KCl is mainly found within the cells of the body.

Other sources of chloride include the following:

- Olives
- Rye flour
- Kelp
- Lettuce
- Tomatoes
- Celery

There is a lot of chloride in seawater; however it is not recommended for consumption as the sodium chloride level in sea water is much too high to drink and it can cause both hypernatremia and hyperchloremia. Chloride does not have to be taken as a supplement as it can be found in most foods we eat on a daily basis, unless you consume a very low salt diet. In such cases, chloride would be supplemented with potassium chloride, which is the main salt substitute found on the market.

23.Testing for Chloride in the blood and Urine

Because chloride is such an essential part of health and living, it is often measured as part of an electrolyte profile, a common blood test performed on the body. A urine test can measure the amount of chloride leaving the body through kidney filtration. In order to do this test, all of the urine excreted during a twenty-four hour period of time is collected and the sodium chloride content of the urine is assessed. The levels of potassium, bicarbonate, sodium, and chloride are usually measured from the bloodstream at the same time in order to get an idea of the electrolyte milieu of the body's bloodstream. Chloride can be measured in a special test called the skin sweat test, in which a patch is placed on the arm for a period of time and the electrolytes in the sweat on the patch are measured. This is a test for cystic fibrosis.

24.Normal Values of Chloride in the Body

The normal reference range for chloride varies with age. For example, a normal chloride content in adult blood is 96-106 mEq/L, while newborn infants can have a chloride content in their blood plasma of between 96 and 113 mEq/L. Adults secrete about 140-250 mEq per 24 hour sample in the urine per 24 hours if they have healthy kidney function. Children and toddlers excrete lesser amounts of chloride in the urine, in the range of 15-176 mEq/24 hour sample.

Remember that chloride concentrations go along directly with the levels of sodium and potassium levels as they are found in dissolved form of NaCl and KCl in the body. For this reason, tests of chloride are rarely done alone but are performed in conjunction with the potassium, sodium, and bicarbonate levels of the blood in a chemistry profile. More information can be retrieved from an entire electrolyte panel than can be done by doing electrolyte levels separate from one another.

Chapter 6:
Potassium

Potassium is a necessary mineral and is very important ion in the body. Potassium is of the class of mineral ions, along with sodium, magnesium, calcium, bicarbonate and chloride; it is essential for life in the human body as well as other animals.

Potassium plays a role in the function of skeletal and smooth muscle, including that of the heart and digestive system. As an electrolyte, it conducts electricity, crucial to intercellular communication.

About 98 percent of all potassium is found within the cells. A proper balance of potassium in the cells and sodium outside of the cells is made possible by pumps within the cellular membranes that exchange sodium and potassium, keeping more potassium in the cells.

High potassium is known as hyperkalemia, while low potassium is called hypokalemia. A simple blood test can determine the level of potassium in the blood plasma. Rarely is the potassium checked alone because more information about the electrolyte content of the blood by testing potassium along with sodium, chloride and CO_2 levels together.

25. Uses of Potassium in the Body

The body needs potassium for the function of every cell in the body. These are main functions of potassium:

- Potassium is important in heartbeat regularity

- Potassium levels help determine the blood pressure

- Potassium is important in muscle contraction, including skeletal and smooth muscles Potassium balance is largely controlled by the kidneys, which remove excess potassium through the urine. A normal level of potassium in plasma (the liquid part of blood) is about 3.5 to 5.0 mEq/L. Notice how small this number is when compared to sodium levels, which are high in the bloodstream and low in the cells. The reverse is true with potassium.

26.Causes of Hypokalemia

Hypokalemia is a common problem. It is estimated that nearly one in five persons hospitalized in the US has a potassium level lower than 3.5 mEq/L. The main causes of low potassium include the following conditions:

- Bulimia
- Anorexia nervosa
- The use of diuretic medications
- Bariatric surgery
- Alcoholism
- AIDS patients
- Diarrhea
- Laxative abuse
- Acute or chronic kidney failure
- Low magnesium levels
- Cushing's syndrome
- Leukemia
- Vomiting
- Following an ileostomy

- Steroid use
- Theophylline use
- Overuse of bronchodilators in asthma management
- Taking loop diuretics like Lasix and Bumex
- Taking antacids excessively
- Taking Diflucan for fungal infections

It should be noted that low potassium can increase your chances of getting digoxin toxicity. Digoxin is used to treat heart failure and, while it doesn't cause low potassium levels, low levels of potassium can increase the risk of digoxin toxicity. Potassium levels are often checked in people taking digoxin for that very reason.

27. Symptoms of Hypokalemia

Hypokalemia can be a silent disease, with no or few symptoms. Some symptoms of low potassium include:

- Tingling and/or numbness of the extremities
- Leg or arm muscle cramping
- Fatigue and weakness
- Nausea and/or vomiting
- Constipation
- Extreme thirst along with an increase in urination
- Low blood pressure
- Fainting
- Psychiatric disturbances, such as delirium, psychosis, hallucinations, and confusion
- Heart palpitations

28.Treatment of Hypokalemia

When treating yourself for low potassium levels, you need to avoid any type of heavy physical activity because potassium is lost from the body during sweating. Avoid the use of diuretics, laxatives and any herbal substances that are known to cause hypokalemia. If you suspect you have potassium deficiency, seek a doctor's advice to see what your potassium level is and to get advice or medication to control the potassium level in the body.

Potassium levels can be brought up by using intravenous or oral medications. Care must be taken when increasing the potassium levels by IV means because it is easy to overshoot the target and cause hyperkalemia. Hyperkalemia can cause severe heart beat abnormalities so that anyone getting potassium replaced needs to be placed on a cardiac monitor which can tell if an abnormal beat has occurred. IV replacement of potassium should be reserved for potassium levels less than mEq/L. Returning the potassium level to normal levels needs to be done as slowly as possible to allow for shifts in potassium and water levels within and outside of the cells and so as to prevent heart problems associated with having a high potassium levels.

When a doctor prescribes oral potassium replacement for low potassium levels, the potassium should be rechecked every two to three days until the potassium levels normalize. If the cause of the hypokalemia is due to the use of a diuretic, you may need to switch to a potassium-sparing diuretic or combine a potassium-sparing diuretic with a potassium-losing diuretic for high blood pressure or fluid retention.

29.Preventing Low Potassium Conditions

If you are at risk for low potassium, there are good food sources of potassium, particularly in the following fruits, meats and vegetables:

· Tomatoes

· Cantaloupes

· Bananas

- Oranges
- Peaches
- Potatoes
- Avocados
- Flounder
- Lima beans
- Chicken
- Cod or salmon

If you are at risk for hypokalemia, you should have your potassium checked every 3-6 months and sooner if you have symptoms of low potassium.

30. Hyperkalemia

In some ways, hyperkalemia or "high potassium" is more dangerous than hypokalemia because high levels of potassium can cause heart arrhythmias and sudden death. The main causes of hyperkalemia include the use of potassium-sparing diuretics and kidney failure. If your kidneys are not working, potassium will not be properly excreted and the potassium level will rise. Addison's disease, in which low levels of aldosterone are in the system, the potassium level will rise to above normal levels.

- There are many different medications that can cause elevated potassium levels. Consider these as possible causes if a patient has high potassium levels and are on any of these medications:
- Antibiotics, like trimethoprim or penicillin
- ACE inhibitors for high blood pressure
- Medications for yeast infections, particularly the azole type medications
- Heparin, for thinning the blood
- NSAIDS, for fever and pain from inflammation

- Herbal supplements such as Siberian ginseng, milkweed, Hawthorn berries, lily of the valley and ground toad skin preparations
- Supplements containing potassium
- Potassium-sparing diuretics, including spironolactone and triamterene

31.Symptoms of Hyperkalemia

The major symptoms of hyperkalemia include the possibility of life threatening heart arrhythmias, bradycardia (slow heart rate) and muscle weakness. If the potassium level is not yet dangerously high, you may have no symptoms at all. A simple lab test can confirm the diagnosis of hyperkalemia. As always, potassium levels are best interpreted in light of checking other electrolytes at the same time. An EKG can show changes consistent with markedly elevated levels of potassium in the bloodstream.

32.Treatment of High Potassium Levels

If the potassium level is extremely high, you need to consider medication that helps reduce the total body amount of potassium. These include the following:

- Diuretics that promote potassium loss in the urine
- IV glucose and insulin, which fills the cells with potassium as well
- Sodium polystyrene sulfonate, which gets rid of potassium through the GI tract
- Kidney dialysis
- Calcium infusion by IV to correct heart rhythm abnormalities

33.Benefits of Potassium

Diets high in potassium have been found to improve bone density among older women. People who are deficient in potassium seem to have higher blood pressure than those who have enough potassium in their system. Potassium in the diet is related to stroke prevention. People with Crohn's disease or ulcerative colitis don't absorb potassium as well as normal people so that they often need potassium supplementation.

34.Taking Potassium supplements

You should always talk to your doctor to see if you need potassium supplementation. There are side effects to taking potassium, such as irritation of the stomach, abnormal heart rate and diarrhea. If you take enough potassium to cause high potassium levels (for example, you should not take potassium supplements if you have kidney failure) you can develop muscle weakness, abnormal rhythms of the heart or bradycardia (slow heart beat). Those who take ACE inhibitors, Bactrim, Septra, or potassium-sparing diuretics, should not take potassium supplementation. The same is true for those who take NSAIDs for inflammation or pain. Beta blocker medication can raise potassium levels.

Chapter 7: Magnesium

Magnesium is actually a common mineral in the body; it is used frequently as a cofactor in more than 300 cellular reactions within the cells. Magnesium is important in energy production, glycolysis, blood sugar control, protein synthesis, muscle function, blood pressure regulation and nerve production. Magnesium is essential for bone health and is an essential cofactor in DNA and RNA synthesis. Magnesium is necessary to run the pumps involved in the transportation of potassium ions and calcium ions into and out of the cells. This is extremely necessary in muscle contraction, the maintenance of heart rhythm, and the conduction of nerve impulses.

At any given point in time, our body contains about 25 grams of magnesium of which more than fifty percent is found in bone. The rest, around 40-50 percent is found in the soft tissue cells with only one percent residing in serum. The normal range of magnesium in a blood test of serum reveals an average value of 0.75 to 0.95 mmol/L. Any number lower than 0.75 mmol/L is considered hypomagnesemia and any number above 0.95 percent is considered to be hypermagnesemia. The homeostasis of magnesium occurs primarily through proper kidney function, which excretes about 120 mg of magnesium daily. If the magnesium levels are low, the kidneys will hold onto more magnesium in order to achieve homeostasis.

Because the vast majority of magnesium is sequestered in soft tissue and bone, the absolute amount of magnesium is difficult to determine with just a blood test. One of the best tests in assessing the total body levels of magnesium is to give a dose of magnesium by IV and to assess the level of magnesium in the urine after that. If the magnesium content of the urine is low despite receiving a bolus of magnesium, it is likely that there are low levels of magnesium in the body.

The recommended dietary allowances or RDAs for magnesium vary with age. For example, in small infants, the RDA for magnesium is only 30 grams per day, while in adults the RDA is between 310 mg and 420 mg per day. Men require more magnesium than women.

35.Magnesium Sources

Ideally we should get our magnesium through the food we eat, although some people would benefit from magnesium supplementation. Great sources of magnesium are legumes, almonds, spinach and other greens, seeds, whole grains and other nuts. Food high in fiber tends also to be high in magnesium. Certain bottled waters and even tap water can be good sources of magnesium intake. Of the magnesium we take into our bodies, only about 30-40 percent is actually absorbed by the gastrointestinal tract.

You can purchase magnesium supplements in the form of a magnesium salt made as magnesium citrate, magnesium oxide and magnesium chloride. When reading the label, the magnesium amount is the weight of the magnesium alone and not the weight of the magnesium salt in the supplement. Magnesium citrate, magnesium lactate, magnesium chloride and magnesium aspartate are particular magnesium supplements that are readily bioavailable once taken in. High zinc intake can interfere with the absorption of magnesium.

Certain laxatives contain high doses of magnesium such as Phillip's Milk of Magnesia®. Certain heartburn medications also contain a great deal of magnesium. Rolaids® is an example of a high source of magnesium.

36.Low Magnesium Levels

Hypomagnesemia is relatively rare due to the ability of the kidneys to hold onto magnesium in times of low magnesium intake. Chronic alcoholism, on the other hand, represents a state of chronically low magnesium and this is a situation where supplemental magnesium needs to be considered.

Signs and symptoms of magnesium deficiency include nausea and vomiting, fatigue and weakness, and poor appetite. Severe hypomagnesemia can cause paresthesias (tingling and numbness) of the extremities, muscle cramps, abnormal heart rhythms, seizures and changes in personality. When the intake of magnesium is low and the blood levels are low, one will also find similar disruptions of calcium and potassium in the bloodstream.

Risk factors for hypomagnesemia include type 2 diabetics, GI diseases that interfere with mineral absorption, alcoholics, the elderly and those with kidney dysfunction. Low levels of potassium can lead to the development of certain diseases, including high blood pressure, osteoporosis, heart disease, type 2 diabetes, and migraines. Magnesium supplementation seems to decrease the risk of sudden cardiovascular death. Stroke is also decreased in those people who have high magnesium levels and type 2 diabetes risk is directly associated with low magnesium levels in the blood. An intake of about 100 mg of magnesium per day has been found to reduce the incidence of type 2 diabetes by 15 percent.

Magnesium is a necessary part of bone growth, influencing the activities of osteoclasts and osteoblasts. Magnesium content affects the parathyroid gland and the amount of vitamin D in the system—both of which regulate the homeostasis of bone growth and mineral content. Some studies have linked low magnesium levels with an increased risk of osteoporosis.

Magnesium loss or poor intake of magnesium is related to the formation of migraine headaches. While this is true, magnesium supplementation doesn't always treat or reduce the number of migraine headaches a person has. Some researchers recommend magnesium intakes of 600 mg per day in divided doses can prevent frequent migraine headaches.

37.High Magnesium Levels

While you can't really suffer from a high magnesium level when you get magnesium from foods, certain supplements, when taken in excess, can raise magnesium levels above the normal range.

High dose magnesium from medications or supplements can lead to crampy abdominal pain, nausea, vomiting, and diarrhea. The laxative effects of magnesium salts are believed to be due to the osmotic effect of having so much magnesium salt in the colon. High magnesium levels also increase gastric motility. Magnesium toxicity can rarely be fatal, especially among the very young and the very old. The risk of hypermagnesemia is highest in those who suffer from renal dysfunction (kidney failure) so that the kidneys fail to get rid of excess magnesium in the diet.

38.Medication Interactions

Magnesium supplementation strongly affects the efficacy of certain medications. For example, magnesium can interfere with the absorption of medications used to treat osteoporosis, primarily the bisphosphonate-type medications, the absorption of tetracycline, the absorption of quinolone antibiotics, proton pump inhibitors like Nexium® and Prevacid®. Magnesium loss can be found when a person takes diuretics such as Lasix® or hydrochlorothiazide in excess for long periods of time.

39.Dietary Intake of Magnesium

Magnesium can come from eating a healthier diet. For example, magnesium can be taken in when eating a wide variety of fruits and vegetables along with whole grains and milk products. Spinach contains high levels of magnesium and certain breakfast cereals will be supplemented with magnesium. Meat, poultry, eggs, nuts, beans and fish are high in magnesium and make for good magnesium levels in the body. Soybeans and legumes like peanuts, lentils and baked beans are high in magnesium. Whole grains in the form of millet and brown rice contain adequate amounts of magnesium as well.

Chapter 8: Calcium

Calcium is the most common form of mineral in the body with the vast majority of calcium being in the bones and teeth (99 percent). Calcium is also used for proper functioning of the nerves, the heart, the muscles, and other body symptoms.

Calcium isn't absorbed nor is it used well if not for the concomitant presence of phosphorus, magnesium, vitamin K and vitamin D. While calcium supplements are plentiful, the best source of absorbable calcium is through the food you eat. Calcium intake is especially important among young children who are continually growing bones and teeth, as well as in pregnant women. Calcium supplements are generally reserved for the following groups of people:

· People who use a lot of caffeine
· Heavy alcohol drinkers
· Postmenopausal women
· Soda drinkers
· Those who take corticosteroids

40.Purposes of Calcium in the Body

Calcium plays a large role in bone formation and maintenance. Bone loss accelerates after age thirty so that by the time a person is elderly, osteoporosis is more common. Bone loss can be prevented by supplementing the diet with calcium and vitamin D. People who have lost their parathyroid glands due to thyroid surgery suffer

Chase Hassen

from low calcium and phosphorus and should take a calcium and vitamin D supplement. They should also refrain from taking in too much phosphorus. Women who suffer from premenstrual syndrome have been found to reduce their symptoms when they take 1,200 mg of calcium per day. This reduces the physical symptoms of PMS, such as bloating, mood disturbances, headache, and food cravings.

Those who suffer from low body calcium levels seem to be at a higher risk of developing high blood pressure. This has been shown in several studies although it is not known if calcium supplementation would turn around high blood pressure on its own. Calcium may prevent high blood pressure in people predisposed to the condition. There have been studies linking high dose calcium intake (up to 2000 mg per day) can reduce their cholesterol levels. Rickets, while rare now, is a disease linked to not getting enough calcium in the diet. People at risk for stroke may benefit from taking a calcium supplement and there is some evidence that calcium along with vitamin D is preventative against colon cancer.

41.Causes of Low Calcium

The most common cause of low calcium is hypoparathyroidism. Everyone has four tiny parathyroid glands imbedded in the thyroid gland. If the thyroid gland has to be removed for any reason and if the parathyroid glands go with it, there can be problems with low calcium and high phosphorus levels.

There is an autoimmune variant of hypoparathyroidism in which antibodies are made against the calcium-sensing receptors in the parathyroid glands. A person can also be born with a congenital defect involving the calcium-sensing receptors. Another hereditary condition causing low calcium is DiGeorge syndrome, in which the parathyroid glands fail to develop.

Low magnesium levels affect the parathyroid hormones and very high magnesium levels lead to an inhibition of parathyroid hormone so that the calcium level may be low. Vitamin D and calcium deficiency combined will result in low calcium levels. Phosphate administration will lower calcium concentrations and acute pancreatitis allows for the deposition of calcium in the abdomen so less calcium is available in the bloodstream. Metastatic cancer (particularly from the breast and prostate gland) will lower the blood calcium levels. Several types of chemotherapy will lower blood calcium levels as well.

42.Signs and Symptoms of Hypocalcemia

If the hypocalcemia is of a gradual onset or is mild, there may be no symptoms at all. If there is a sudden or severe loss of calcium, the patient may suffer from tetany of the muscles and hyperactivity of the nerves. There can be numbness or tingling sensations of the fingertips and around the mouth. People with low calcium levels can suffer from muscle cramps. Breathing can be affected if the muscles required for breathing are in spasm. Other symptoms of low calcium include:

· Dementia or mental retardation

· Seizure activity

· Anxiety or depression

· Parkinson's symptoms

· Brain calcifications

· Increased muscular irritability

· Low blood pressure or heart failure

· Sweating

· Asthma symptoms (bronchospasm)

43.Diagnosing Low Calcium

A person is said to have hypocalcemia if they have a total serum calcium level of less than 8.2 mg/dL or an ionized level lower than 4.4 mg/dL. The physical examination may show some of the signs noted above. Patients who have chronic kidney disease or who lost their parathyroid gland function are all at risk for low calcium concentration in the blood.

44.Treatment of Hypocalcemia

Treatment of hypocalcemia can benefit from IV replacement with calcium gluconate. The first 1-2 grams of calcium gluconate should be given slowly over 10-20 minutes as too rapidly replacing calcium can affect heart rhythm. Calcium can irritate the veins so it should be highly diluted in normal saline or dextrose solutions. Check the magnesium level in all patients with low calcium because the two can go together and magnesium may need to be replaced as well. Replacement should be slow and gradual especially in patients who suffer from kidney damage. Calcium is often given along with vitamin D for maximum effectiveness. Diuretic therapy can also increase the kidneys' abilities to hang onto calcium.

45.Signs and Symptoms of High Calcium Levels

With high calcium levels, there can be overworking of the kidneys, leading to thirstiness and frequent urination. You can get abdominal pain, nausea, vomiting, or constipation from high calcium levels. The excess calcium in the bloodstream usually comes from a leaching of calcium out of the bones, so you can get bony pain and osteoporosis. You can have weakness of the muscles and brain symptoms such as confusion, fatigue and malaise.

46.Calcium Supplementation

The best dietary sources of calcium come from dairy products, including milk, cheeses and yogurt. Blackstrap molasses and tofu are rich in calcium. Certain nuts, cabbage, broccoli, kelp and dark leafy greens contain a great deal of calcium as well. Non-plant sources of calcium include fortified cereals, salmon, oysters and sardines.

You can buy calcium supplements with or without vitamin D. Calcium citrate is the easiest to absorb when compared to calcium carbonate; however, the latter is cheaper to buy. Calcium carbonate should be taken with orange juice or other acidic drink because this helps the calcium to absorb better.

The dose of calcium supplements vary with age. Newborns and infants should receive about 200 mg per day, while adults up to age

50 need 1000 mg per day. Women who are postmenopausal may need up to 1,200 mg of calcium daily.

There are side effects whenever you take calcium supplements. This can include constipation, stomach indigestion, confusion, renal failure, and irregular heartbeats. If you have hyperparathyroidism, cancer, kidney failure or sarcoidosis, you shouldn't take calcium by means of supplementation and should get calcium strictly from the diet.

Calcium supplementation should be taken under the care of your doctor if you are taking bisphosphonates such as Fosamax® or Didronel®. Aluminum containing antacids can cause an elevated absorption of calcium citrate. Blood pressure medications like beta-blockers and calcium channel blockers can be interfered with if you take calcium supplementation.

People on digoxin for heart failure may experience toxicity to digoxin, while low levels of calcium interfere with the activity of digoxin. Thiazide diuretics can raise the calcium level in the bloodstream, while loop diuretics like Lasix® can reduce calcium levels. Calcium supplements can block quinolone antibiotic absorption and tetracycline absorption. Dilantin® and other seizure medication can reduce serum calcium levels.

Chapter 9:
Phosphorus

Phosphorus is the second most common mineral found in the human body, just behind calcium. Phosphorus is essential for proper health; it is used in enzymatic reactions that grow and repair tissues of the body. A total of 85 percent of the phosphorus in the body is found in your bones and teeth, providing strong bones and teeth.

47.Purposes of Phosphorus

The phosphorus molecule is found inside the body as the phosphate ion. Phosphates are essential to making ATP, which is the main energy molecule in the body. The phosphorus in ATP is lost during an energy reaction in which ATP (adenosine triphosphate) turns into ADP (adenosine diphosphate), releasing energy to power cellular reactions.

Phosphorus is also a major component of DNA and RNA in the cells. Without phosphorus, we would have no genetic blueprint within the cells. If we don't get enough phosphorus, protein synthesis is impaired and the cells of the body suffer.

Phosphorus is a natural buffer which acts to neutralize acids in the body so that the pH is kept at 7.4. The hemoglobin in our bloodstream and many bodily enzymes make use of phosphorus as a cofactor or as a part of the structure of the protein itself.

48.Where do you get phosphorus in the diet?

Much of the phosphorus in our diet comes from a wide variety of foods, such as eggs, milk, fish, legumes, grains and cereals. Carbonated beverages of any type contain a lot of phosphorus, even though they are not always healthful in other ways. Food additives also have a great deal of phosphorus in them. It is recommended that we take in about 700 mg of phosphorus daily. Amounts of phosphorus exceeding 4 grams per day are not healthy for you so you should watch your phosphorus intake, especially if you have kidney problems. The calcium intake in your diet should roughly match the amount of phosphorus in your diet because bones and teeth require equal amounts of these minerals. It is rare to have a phosphorus deficiency because it is so plentiful in the diet.

49.Low Phosphorus Levels

Certain medications, such as antacids and diuretics, can cause a reduction in the serum phosphorus content. Other conditions can result in a low phosphorus content, such as type 2 diabetes, alcoholism, and starvation. Diseases of the bowel such as celiac disease and Crohn's disease can be so severe as to limit the amount of phosphorus and other minerals absorbed by the GI tract. In such cases, the phosphorus levels can be too low.

If the phosphorus level is too low, some symptoms can be anxiety, bony pain, lack of appetite, osteoporosis, fatigue, joint stiffness, numbness, irritability, breathing problems and weight fluctuations. Children with low phosphorus levels do not grow properly because they need phosphorus for healthy bone growth and teeth formation.

50.High Phosphorus Content

Too much phosphorus in the bloodstream happens more commonly that low phosphorus situations. High phosphorus can be because of kidney disease, taking too much phosphorus in the diet or consuming too little calcium, which must balance out with the amount of phosphorus you take in. High phosphorus levels are linked to an increase in cardiovascular disease risk. Too much phosphate in your system can lead to phosphorus toxicity, leading to diarrhea and hardening of the arteries (atherosclerosis). Too much phosphate can also lead to an interference with the ability of the body to use calcium, zinc, magnesium and iron. Some athletes take phosphorus before strenuous activity to prevent muscle stiffness. This should only be done under a doctor's care so that the phosphorus level doesn't get too high.

Ideally, there should be a balance between the calcium and phosphorus intake in the body. Unfortunately, modern western diets contain a great deal more phosphorus than calcium and calcium must be leached from bones and teeth in order to match the amount of phosphorus in the bloodstream; the bones can become brittle.

Chapter 10:
Conclusion

It is a serious understatement to say that electrolytes are necessary for life. Electrolytes are charged mineral particles that create the environment of our cells and our interstitial fluid. Sodium and potassium, along with chloride and bicarbonate, set the stage for the environmental milieu and keep the amount of water in the various body compartments as stable as possible.

Minerals ions are used as cofactors in enzymatic reactions that are part of cellular metabolism. They can also be used as part of the enzymes themselves. Phosphorus, for example, is a big part of cellular ATP, used to create the energy needed for cellular functions. Phosphorus also makes up the substance of our nuclear material, such as DNA and the various types of RNA.

Much of the electrolyte balance in our bodies is determined by the kidneys, which filter electrolytes and respond to changes in electrolyte concentration of the blood by holding onto or excreting electrolytes in order to maintain proper electrolyte concentrations in the body. If you suffer from kidney failure, the electrolytes do not balance properly and there can be excesses or deficiencies of certain electrolytes.

Electrolyte balance is a big part of homeostasis in the body. There is, by necessity, more potassium in the cells than in the bloodstream and more sodium in the bloodstream than in the cells. This homeostasis is managed by potassium and sodium pumps that create the marked difference between the intracellular milieu and the extracellular milieu.

Most diets contain enough of the various electrolytes, with the exception of possibly calcium. The intake of phosphorus should ideally keep up with the intake of calcium as they are used in equal quantities in bones and teeth. Unfortunately, Western diets are much too high in phosphorus intake when compared to calcium intake so that calcium is leached from the bone in order to maintain bloodstream concentrations of calcium and phosphorus that are equal to one another. This can lead to brittle bones.

Electrolytes create an environment in which the enzymes can work properly for all the various reactions necessary for health. The cellular and extracellular quantities of the various electrolytes determine the pH of these tissue areas so that enzymatic processes can happen in the proper pH range.

If you enjoyed this book, would you be kind enough to leave a review on Amazon? Your positive reviewers can help others to see what kinds of helpful resources are out there!

If you would like to be updated when each one of my new books come out, I will send you an email when it goes on free promotion! Just Click Here. I'll talk to you soon and see you in the next book!

Thank you and good luck on your medical endeavors!

NCLEX: Fluids, Electrolytes & Acid Base Disorders

105 Nursing Practice Questions and Rationales to Absolutely Crush the NCLEX!

Chase Hassen

Nurse Superhero

© 2015

Disclaimer:

Although the author and publisher have made every effort to ensure that the information in this book was correct at press time, the author and publisher do not assume and hereby disclaim any liability to any party for any loss, damage, or disruption caused by errors or omissions, whether such errors or omissions result from negligence, accident, or any other cause.

This book is not intended as a substitute for the medical advice of physicians. The reader should regularly consult a physician in matters relating to his/her health and particularly with respect to any symptoms that may require diagnosis or medical attention.

Table of Contents

Chapter 1: NCLEX Answers & Rationales on Fluids, Electrolytes, and Acid Base Disorders

The following are the questions on the test you have just taken along with the correct answers and rationales.

1. Why are the elderly more likely to get electrolyte and fluid disorders?

    a. They don't have the drive to drink as much.

    b. They absorb electrolytes more poorly.

    c. The kidneys don't work as well.

    d. Their bodies only contain 45-55 percent water as opposed to 60 percent in young adults.

Answer: d. Because elderly bodies contain a less percentage of water, there is more likely to be fluid imbalances and electrolyte disturbances.

2. The fluid found in the blood vessels is called what?

    a. Intracellular fluid

    b. Interstitial fluid

    c. Transcellular fluid

    d. Intravascular fluid

Answer: d. The fluid or plasma within the blood vessels is called the intravascular fluid space. Intracellular fluid is found within the cells and interstitial fluid is that fluid found around the cells. Transcellular fluid is fluid such as cerebrospinal fluid, pericardial fluid, pleural fluid, and GI secretions.

3. The natural pathway of electrolytes from a high concentration to a lower concentration is called what?

   a. Facilitated diffusion

   b. Diffusion

   c. Active transport

   d. Osmosis

Answer: b. Diffusion is the natural pathway of electrolytes from a high concentration to a lower concentration. It involves no facilitated or active processes. Osmosis is fluid transport across a membrane.

4. Movement of a molecule across a selectively permeable membrane against a normal concentration gradient requires what?

   a. Diffusion

   b. Active transport

   c. Facilitated diffusion

   d. Osmosis

Answer: b. Active transport involves energy that takes a molecule against a concentration gradient across a selectively permeable membrane.

5. Movement of water and its solutes from an area of high hydrostatic pressure to an area of low hydrostatic pressure is called what?

   a. Active transport

   b. Facilitated transport

   c. Filtration

   d. Osmosis

Answer: c. Filtration is the movement of water and solutes from an area of high hydrostatic pressure to an area of lower hydrostatic pressure.

6. The receptors for thirst are disrupted in a client. Where in the client's body is this disruption occurring?

   a. Peripheral blood pressure sensors

   b. Hypothalamus

   c. Pituitary gland

   d. Adrenal glands

Answer: b. The centers for thirst are located within the hypothalamus and are stimulated by low blood pressure and elevated serum osmolality.

7. A concerned client asks how much urine is produced by the kidneys in an average day. How do you answer?

   a. About a liter a day

   b. 100 cc per hour

   c. 1.5 liters per day

   d. 3 liters per day

Answer: c. An average amount of urine produced per day is about 30 cc per hour or about 1.5 liters per day. Of course, the actual amount of urine put out per day depends largely on intake.

8. Hormones important in the regulation of fluid and electrolyte balance include these. Select all that apply.

   a. Renin

   b. Angiotensin

   c. Antidiuretic hormone (ADH)

   d. Aldosterone

   e. Cortisol

   f. ACTH

Answer: c. d. Both ADH and aldosterone regulate the fluid and electrolyte balance through their action on the kidneys.

9. How much fluid is secreted and reabsorbed by the GI tract every day?

   a. 200 cc

   b. 1-2 liter

   c. 3-4 liters

   d. 6-8 liters

Answer: c. The GI tract secretes and resorbs about 3-4 liters of fluid per day, leaving only less than 250 cc in the gut at the end of the digestive process to be passed into the stool.

10. What primarily causes fluid to stay in the intravascular space?

   a. Immunoglobulins

   b. Albumin

   c. Osmosis

   d. Active transport of water from the intracellular spaces

Answer: b. Albumin and other lesser proteins are responsible for keeping fluid in the intravascular space. Albumin is the most abundant intravascular protein.

11. Angiotensin II inhibitors decrease blood pressure by what mechanism?

   a. It lessens the renin produced by the kidneys.

   b. It reduces the production of aldosterone.

c. It acts to have less vasoconstriction.

d. It directly decreases resorption of sodium in the kidneys.

Answer: c. Angiotensin II inhibitors block vasoconstriction, reducing blood pressure.

12. The actions of aldosterone on the kidneys are what? Select all that apply.

    a. Increases sodium excretion.

    b. Increases potassium excretion

    c. Increase hydrogen ion excretion

    d. Decreases sodium excretion

    e. Increases water resorption

    f. Decreases water resorption

Answer: b. c. d. Aldosterone increases the excretion of potassium ions and hydrogen ions while causing the reabsorption of sodium into the system. Water follows the absorption of sodium.

13. What hormone is responsible for the absorption of water from the kidneys back into the system?

    a. Antidiuretic hormone

    b. Angiotensin II

    c. Renin

    d. Aldosterone

Answer: a. Antidiuretic hormone or ADH is secreted by the hypothalamus and is responsible for the reabsorption of water from the kidneys.

14. Hypotonic IV solutions are given in what type of situation?

    a. Hypotonic dehydration

    b. Blood transfusions

    c. GI losses of fluid

    d. Hyponatremia

Answer: c. Hypotonic IV solution is given in situations of GI fluid losses, hypertonic dehydration and after normal saline fluid resuscitation in diabetic acidosis if the glucose is still greater than 250.

15. Which IV solution is contraindicated in renal and liver insufficiency?

    a. Lactated Ringer's solution

    b. Normal Saline

    c. D5W and half normal saline

    d. 10 percent dextrose

Answer: a. Lactated Ringer's solution is contraindicated in situations of renal or liver insufficiency. It is similar to serum and cannot be given in cases of a blood pH of greater than 7.5.

16. What is the purpose of giving a colloidal solution to the client?

    a. To correct a hyponatremic state.

    b. To expand blood volume.

c. To treat diabetic ketoacidosis.

d. To treat hypotonic states.

Answer: b. Colloidal fluids have cells, proteins, or large molecules in them that help expand blood volume. They keep fluid within the intravascular space.

17. What is the major cation in extracellular fluid?

    a. Potassium

    b. Sodium

    c. Chloride

    d. Magnesium

Answer: b. Sodium is the major cation in extracellular fluid while potassium is the major cation in intracellular fluid. Chloride is the major anion (negatively charged particle) in extracellular fluid.

18. What are the major functions of intracellular potassium? Select all that apply.

    a. Maintains intracellular sodium concentration at a low level.

    b. Conducts nerve impulses

    c. Contracts myocardium, skeletal muscle, and smooth muscle

    d. Provides enzymatic action for cellular energy production

    e. Regulates osmolality of intracellular fluid

    f. Regulates osmolality of extracellular fluid

Answer: b. c. d. e. Potassium helps conduct nerve impulses and helps to contract muscular cells of all types. It also provides support for cellular energy production and regulates the osmolality of intracellular fluid.

19. Which cation is most responsible for acid base balance in the extracellular fluid?

    a. HCO3-

    b. Na+

    c. K+

    d. Cl-

Answer: b. Sodium (Na+) can bind with HCO3- or Cl-, thereby controlling the acid base balance in the extracellular fluid.

20. The bulk of Phosphorus in the form of phosphate can be found in what body area?

    a. Bones

    b. Bone marrow

    c. Teeth

    d. Serum

Answer: a. Phosphorus is found mostly in bones and teeth; however, as there are more bony areas than teeth, phosphorus is mainly found in bones, combined with calcium.

21. A normal blood pH is between_____ and

    _____.

Answer: 7.35, 7.45

_____

22. A client has a blood pH of 7.3. You know that this represents what?

   a. Alkalosis

   b. Normal pH value

   c. Acidosis

   d. Neutral pH value

Answer: c. A client with a blood pH of 7.3 is suffering from acidosis.

23. A client is suffering from respiratory failure and has an excess of CO_2. What condition is the client suffering from?

   a. Metabolic acidosis

   b. Metabolic alkalosis

   c. Respiratory acidosis

   d. Respiratory alkalosis

Answer: c. Underbreathing causes an excess of CO_2, which contributes to acidosis. Because the cause is respiratory, the client is suffering from respiratory acidosis.

24. What would the client's respiratory response be to a low CO_2 level?

   a. Increase rate of respiration.

   b. Increase depth of respiration.

   c. Decrease respiratory center stimulation

   d. Decrease rate and depth of breaths

Answer: d. The client would decrease rate and depth of breaths in order to hold onto more CO_2.

25. In cases of blood acidosis or alkalosis, what is the first response to alter the pH balance?

    a. A change in respiratory rate

    b. A change in renal excretion of acids or bases

    c. Sodium attaches to Cl- or HCO3- inside the cells

    d. Potassium is shunted outside the cells.

Answer: a. Renal responses to changes in pH can take hours to days and changes sodium binding do not appreciably affect pH in the cells. Potassium shifts do not appreciably change extracellular pH. Therefore, the first response to alkalosis or acidosis is to change the respiratory function.

26. How does the kidney respond to pH increases in the bloodstream?

    a. It holds onto NaHCO3.

    b. It conserves H+ and excretes NaHCO3.

    c. It excretes KOH and holds onto NaHCO3.

    d. It conserves albumin and excretes H+.

Answer: b. In response to a pH decrease, the kidneys hold on to H+ and excrete NaHCO3.

27. A client has a normal urine pH of 6. Why is this so?

    a. It excretes H+ ions more than it excretes bicarbonate.

    b. It excretes albumin, which is acidic.

    c. It excretes acidic by-products of cellular metabolism

    d. It holds onto more CO_2 than HCO_3-.

Answer: c. The kidneys excrete by-products of cellular metabolism, which make the urine acidic.

28. A client has an arterial blood gas with a pH of 7.45. What might this represent?

    a. Compensated alkalosis.

    b. Respiratory acidosis.

    c. Respiratory failure.

    d. Acute hypoventilation.

Answer: a. A client with a blood gas showing a pH likely has a compensated alkalosis. The others represent situations of low pH.

29. In determining whether or not a blood pH of 7.3 represents respiratory acidosis, what part of the blood gas determination should be looked at next?

    a. The HCO_3- level

    b. The $PaCO_2$ level

    c. The ratio of HCO_3- to $PaCO_2$

d. The urinary H+ level

Answer: b. The blood gas PaCO2 level will tell you whether or not a pH of 7.3 is respiratory acidosis or not. If it is elevated, the person likely has respiratory acidosis because CO2 brings down the blood pH.

30. The metabolic component of acid-base balance in a client is what?

    a. Albumin concentration

    b. PaCO2 level

    c. HCO3- level

    d. NaOH level

Answer: c. The metabolic component of acid-base balance is the HCO3- level. This is determined by the kidney's response to changes in pH.

31. You are trying to determine if there is a primary metabolic pH problem in the client. What do you look for?

    a. Lactic acid levels

    b. That the pH and HCO3- levels go in the same direction.

    c. That the pH and HCO3- levels are reciprocal.

    d. That the PaCO2 level is unaffected.

Answer: b. As long as the pH and HCo3- are going in the same direction, the patient has a primary metabolic problem.

32. A normal PaCO2 level is what?

    a. 10-12 mmHg

    b. 15-20 mmHg

    c. 20-30 mmHg

d.   35-45 mmHg

Answer: d. A normal PaCO2 level is 35-45 mmHg.

33. A client has lost 15 percent of his body weight within 12 hours. What is the client's diagnosis?

    a. Mild hypovolemia

    b. Moderate hypovolemia

    c. Severe hypovolemia

    d. Hypotension

Answer: c. A patient who is suffering from 10-15 percent of body weight loss is suffering from severe hypovolemia.

34. A client is hypotensive, has low urine output and has a normal hemoglobin. What is a possible cause of these symptoms?

    a. Acute hemorrhage

    b. Diarrhea with fluid loss

    c. Vomiting with fluid loss

    d. Kidney failure

Answer: a. With hypotension and a poor urine output, the patient is likely suffering from hypovolemia. The normal hemoglobin supports sudden blood loss as a cause of the hypovolemia.

35. One way to assess whether the patient's hypovolemia is due to renal loss or an extra-renal loss is to do what?

    a. Check a serum creatinine

    b. Check a urine specific gravity

    c. Check a urine creatinine level

    d. Check a BUN/creatinine ratio

Answer: b. If you check a urine specific gravity, it should be high if the dehydration is secondary to an extra-renal cause of the dehydration. If it is low, renal losses of water may be the cause.

36. You are treating a client with dehydration by giving extra fluids. What other nursing intervention would be appropriate?

    a. Put the patient in the Trendelenburg position

    b. Put the patient with legs elevated at 45 degrees

    c. Put the patient in the prone position

    d. Put tourniquets around the thighs to conserve water in the trunk.

Answer: b. The patient should lie supine or have legs elevated to 45 degrees. The Trendelenburg position is contraindicated as it can interfere with breathing.

37. Reasons for hypervolemia could include the following. Select all that apply.

   a. Excessive intake of fluid and sodium.

   b. Chronic renal failure

   c. Diuretic therapy

   d. Excess D5W infusion

   e. Acute renal failure

   f. Potassium loss

Answer: a. b. e. Excess intake of both fluid and sodium, chronic and acute renal failure can all cause hypervolemia.

38. Integumentary signs of hypervolemia include the following. Select all that apply.

   a. Warm extremities

   b. Anasarca

   c. Dependent edema

   d. Eczematoid rash

   e. Gangrenous extremities

Answer: b. c. Common integumentary signs of hypervolemia include cold extremities, anasarca, and dependent edema.

39. A client with hypervolemia has evidence of pulmonary edema. What nursing interventions might be ordered? Select all that apply.

    a. D5W with 0.5 normal saline by IV

    b. IV morphine

    c. Oxygen by mask

    d. Nitroglycerine sublingually

    e. Normal saline

    f. Mannitol by IV

Answer: b. c. d. IV morphine, nitroglycerine and O2 by mask are all appropriate interventions for pulmonary edema. Fluid should be restricted, sodium should be restricted. IV mannitol is used for cerebral edema.

40. Loop diuretics are used to reduce fluid retention in your client. What should you look out for?

    a. Hyperkalemia

    b. Hyponatremia

    c. Hypokalemia

    d. Hypernatremia

Answer: c. Hypokalemia is a side effect of loop diuretic therapy. The other findings are not side effects of loop diuretics. Hyperkalemia is a side effect of potassium-sparing diuretics.

41. Hypokalemia is a serum potassium level less than
_____ mEq/l.

Answer: ____3.5____

42. The client's EKG revealed flattened T waves, depressed ST segment and the presence of a U wave. What electrolyte disturbance do you suspect?

   a. Hyperkalemia

   b. Hypokalemia

   c. Hypernatremia

   d. Hyponatremia

Answer: b. The above EKG findings can be seen in clients with hypokalemia.

43. A client requires urgent replacement of potassium. Which is the best way to give potassium to this client who has a central line?

   a. IV replacement at no greater than 10mEq/hr

   b. Oral K replacement with meals

   c. A bolus of 20 mEq K over 10 minutes

   d. IV replacement of no greater than 20 mEq/hr

Answer: d. IV replacement of potassium can be given at no greater than 10 mEq/hr in peripheral lines and no greater than 20 mEq/hr in a central line. As the client has a central line placed, you can give up to 20 mEq/hr. Potassium cannot be given as a bolus.

44. Hyperkalemia is defined as a serum potassium of greater than_____ mEq/l.

Answer: ___5.0___

45. A client has a serum potassium of 6.4 mEq/l. The complication most feared is what?

    a. Hypotension

    b. Heart block

    c. Neuromuscular irritability

    d. Cardiac arrest

Answer: d. All of the possible are outcomes of hyperkalemia. The most serious of these is cardiac arrest.

46. A client has an EKG showing tall, peaked T waves, a prolonged PR interval, ST depression, flattened P waves and a widened QRS. What metabolic condition do you suspect?

    a. Hypokalemia

    b. Hyponatremia

    c. Hyperphosphatemia

    d. Hyperkalemia

Answer: d. In a client with hyperkalemia, the above EKG changes can be present.

47. The treatment of choice for severe hyperkalemia is what?

    a. Oral or nasogastric Kayexelate

    b. Avoid bananas and spinach

    c. Sorbitol orally

    d. Calcium gluconate 10 percent IV

Answer: a. Oral, rectal, or nasogastric Kayexelate is given as a treatment for severe hyperkalemia. Sometimes oral sorbitol is added to facilitate stool loss of Kayexelate. Avoiding potassium-containing foods is a good idea but not enough to treat elevated potassium levels. Calcium gluconate can counteract the neuromuscular and cardiac effects of elevated potassium but it does not decrease K levels and is only temporary.

48. A client has been diagnosed with SIADH (Syndrome of Inappropriate ADH Secretion. What electrolyte values are correct?

    a. Elevated serum sodium, elevated urine sodium

    b. Decreased serum sodium, elevated urine sodium

    c. Elevated serum sodium, decreased urine sodium

    d. Decreased serum sodium, decreased urine sodium

Answer: b. In SIADH, the serum sodium is decreased and the urine sodium is increased.

49. A client has been diagnosed with diabetes insipidus. The urine osmolality is _____(Increased or

decreased) and the serum sodium is
_____(increased/decreased).

Answer: <u>decreased, increased</u>

_____

50. The main cause of low calcium in any individual is:

    a. Low calcium intake

    b. Low vitamin D intake

    c. Elevated phosphorus levels

    d. Renal failure

Answer: d. The principal cause of hypocalcemia is renal failure. The others can cause low calcium but are less likely.

51. Clinical manifestations of low calcium include the following. Select all that apply.

    a. Tetany

    b. Muscle flaccidity

    c. Negative Trousseau's sign

    d. Positive Chvostek's sign

    e. Shorter clotting times

    f. Skeletal fractures

Answer: a. d. f. Signs of low calcium include tetany and muscular irritability, positive Trousseau's sign, positive Chvostek's sign, longer clotting times and skeletal fractures. VTach and EKG changes can also happen.

52. Why should a serum albumin level be checked along with a serum calcium level?

    a. Because calcium is drawn into bones by elevated albumin levels

    b. Because calcium is carried on albumin and they can rise and fall together

    c. Because albumin draws calcium into cells

    d. Because albumin contains a lot of calcium ions in it

Answer: b. Calcium is carried on the protein, albumin, so if albumin levels are low, so is the total calcium level.

53. An asymptomatic client has low ionized Calcium levels. How is this best treated?

    a. By giving oral calcium supplements

    b. By adding CaCl to the IV Bag

    c. By giving a CaCl IV push

    d. By encouraging milk drinking

Answer: a. An asymptomatic person with low ionized Calcium levels should be treated with oral Calcium supplements. IV calcium is not necessary and milk drinking might be too slow.

54. A patient has low ionized calcium and tetany/arrhythmias. How is this best treated?

    a. Oral calcium supplements

b. Taking in more glasses of milk

c. 10 cc of 10 percent Calcium Gluconate by IV push

d. 15 cc of 10 percent Calcium gluconate over 15 minutes

Answer: d. 10-20 cc of 10 percent Calcium gluconate should be given at 1 cc per minute to avoid hypotension and bradycardia.

55. A risk of giving Calcium by IV is what?

    a. It can reduce the effectiveness of digoxin

    b. It can cause tissue necrosis, especially when given by peripheral IV

    c. It can cause irritability of the muscles

    d. It can cause seizures

Answer: b. Calcium chloride or calcium gluconate can cause tissue necrosis so the IV site should be monitored closely or it should be given centrally.

56. Signs of hypercalcemia include the following. Select all that apply.

    a. Lethargy

    b. Constipation

    c. Confusion

    d. Muscle tetany

    e. Positive Chvostek's sign

    f. Positive Trousseau's sign

Answer: a. c. Signs of hypercalcemia include lethargy, confusion and nausea. The Chvostek's sign and Trousseau's sign are positive in hypocalcemia as is muscle tetany.

57. A major cause of hypercalcemia is what?

   a. Low calcium intake

   b. Elevated albumin in serum

   c. Bone loss of calcium

   d. High phosphate levels

Answer: b. The major cause of hypercalcemia is bone loss of calcium. Low calcium intake is unlikely to cause hypercalcemia and elevated albumin and phosphate levels are unlikely to cause hypercalcemia.

58. A client has a shortened ST segment and shortened QT interval with a prolonged PR interval. What metabolic problem is likely?

   a. Hypocalcemia

   b. Hypercalcemia

   c. Hyperkalemia

   d. Hypokalemia

Answer: b. Hypercalcemia can cause a shortened ST segment, shortened QT interval and a prolonged PR interval.

59. X-ray evidence of hypercalcemia include the following. Select all that apply.

    a. Urinary calculi

    b. Osteoporosis

    c. Increased bone density

    d. Pathological fractures

    e. Mottled bone

    f. Paget's disease of bone

Answer: a. b. d. X-ray evidence of elevated calcium levels include urinary calculi, osteoporosis and pathological fractures. The calcium is mostly in the serum and none of it is in the bones.

60. Nursing interventions for clients with hypercalcemia include the following. Select all that apply.

    a. Drink more milk.

    b. Drink 3-4 liters of fluid per day.

    c. Eat more bananas.

    d. Eat high acid-containing foods.

    e. Take a loop diuretic.

    f. Take a thiazide diuretic.

Answer: b. d. e. Clients with hypercalcemia should drink extra fluids to prevent calculi, eat acid-containing foods to prevent calculi and to take normal saline with a loop diuretic to draw out calcium in the urine.

61. The purpose of IV bisphosphonates in the treatment of hypercalcemia is what?

   a. To increase urinary excretion of calcium.

   b. To increase urinary uptake of calcium from bones

   c. To prevent calcium release from bones.

   d. To decrease urinary calculi in the kidneys and ureters.

Answer: c. Bisphosphonates prevent calcium release from the bones so calcium levels drop naturally.

62. Nursing treatments for severe hypophosphatemia include:

   a. Eat high phosphorus foods.

   b. Give parathyroid hormone.

   c. Give powdered phosphorus supplement

   d. Give IV potassium phosphate via an infusion pump.

Answer: d. IV potassium phosphate slowly via an infusion pump, such as potassium phosphate at 10 mEq/hr.

63. Complications of IV potassium phosphate infusion include the following. Select all that apply.

    a. Tissue necrosis

    b. Hypercalcemia

    c. Hypophosphatemia

    d. Hypocalcemia

    e. Hyperphosphatemia

    f. Muscle weakness

Answer: a. d. e. Complications of IV potassium phosphate infusion include tissue necrosis, hypocalcemia, tetany and hyperphosphatemia.

64. The most common cause of hyperphosphatemia is what?

    a. Dialysis

    b. Renal failure, acute or chronic

    c. Hyperlipidemia

    d. Malignancies

Answer: b. The most common cause of hyperphosphatemia is acute or chronic renal failure. Malignancies are a less common cause of hyperphosphatemia.

65. Low magnesium levels are often due to what?

    a. Elevated calcium levels

    b. Hyperkalemia

    c. Chronic alcoholism

    d. Diabetes insipidus

Answer: c. Common causes of low magnesium are due to chronic alcoholism and uncontrolled diabetes mellitus

66. A client has developed Torsades de pointes. What electrolyte abnormality do you suspect?

    a. Hypomagnesemia

    b. Hypermagnesemia

    c. Hypokalemia

    d. Hyponatremia

Answer: a. Torsades de pointes is often associated with low magnesium levels.

67. A low magnesium level is often associated with what?

    a. Elevated albumin levels

    b. Elevated calcium levels

    c. Low potassium levels

    d. Low calcium levels

Answer: d. Calcium is required for PTH secretion so it may be low in combination with low magnesium levels.

68. Hypermagnesemia is often associated with what condition?

    a. Magnesium-containing antacids

    b. Renal failure with elevated intake of magnesium

    c. Diabetes insipidus

    d. SIADH

Answer: b. Elevated magnesium is often associated with renal failure along with taking in too much magnesium.

69. If the client's magnesium level is too high, a common treatment is what?

    a. Give half normal saline and diuretics.

    b. Provide sodium chloride using normal saline.

    c. Give Potassium chloride by IV.

    d. Give medications to promote stool excretion of magnesium.

Answer: a. Half normal saline and diuretics to promote renal excretion of magnesium. Severe Hypermagnesemia can be treated with 10 percent calcium chloride, 10 cc by IV.

70. The most common cause of respiratory acidosis is:

    a. Hyperventilation

    b. Alveolar hypoventilation

    c. COPD

d. Asthma

Answer: b. Respiratory acidosis is due to alveolar hypoventilation with an acute increase in PaCO2. Hyperventilation results in respiratory alkalosis and COPD is usually well compensated.

71. A drug test should be performed in cases of respiratory acidosis because:

    a. Drugs can increase the acidosis of the body.

    b. Drugs can affect the kidney's ability to hold onto bicarbonate.

    c. Drugs can cause hypoventilation.

    d. Drugs can interfere with alveolar function.

Answer: c. Drugs can interfere with respirations, causing respiratory failure and hypoventilation.

72. Causes of metabolic acidosis include:

    a. Pneumonia

    b. Guillain-Barre syndrome

    c. Narcotics

    d. Diabetic ketoacidosis

Answer: d. Diabetic ketoacidosis is a cause of metabolic acidosis. The others are considered causes of respiratory acidosis.

73. Causes of respiratory alkalosis include the following. Select all that apply.

    a. Anxiety

    b. Narcotics

    c. Asthma

    d. Hyperventilation

    e. Pain

    f. Hypokalemia

Answer: a. d. e. Anxiety, pain, fever, and hyperventilation all can cause respiratory alkalosis. Narcotics cause respiratory acidosis and hypokalemia causes metabolic alkalosis.

74. An intubated client who has unilateral lung disease causing an acid base disorder can benefit from what positioning techniques?

    a. Lie in Trendelenburg position

    b. Lie with feet at 45 degrees elevation

    c. Lie on side with unaffected side up

    d. Lie on side with unaffected side down.

Answer: d. An intubated client can be positioned on the side with the unaffected side down to facilitate respirations and decrease acid-base disorders.

75. Nursing interventions in acid-base disorders include the following:

 a. Look for and treat underlying cause.

 b. Increase or decrease the IV rate.

 c. Give sodium bicarbonate or sodium hydroxide depending on the pH.

 d. Give sedatives or propofol.

Answer: a. The best nursing intervention for acid-base disorders is to treat the underlying cause of the pathology.

76. The respiratory response to metabolic acidosis includes:

 a. Hypoventilation

 b. Bronchospasm

 c. Kussmaul's respirations

 d. Cheyne-Stokes Respirations

Answer: c. As a response to metabolic acidosis, the patient has deep and rapid respirations to blow off CO_2. These are called Kussmaul's respirations.

77. The client has compensated metabolic acidosis. What finding will be noted on ABGs?

 a. Low pH

 b. Increased PCO_2

   c. Normal pH

   d. Elevated urine pH

Answer: c. If the client has compensated metabolic acidosis, the pH will be normal but the PCO2 will be decreased and the urine pH will be decreased in an attempt to normalize the blood pH.

78. Why is the serum K+ increased in metabolic acidosis?

   a. K+ leaks out of cells that are leakier in this situation.

   b. K+ is exchanged for H+ that goes into the cells to normalize blood pH

   c. K+ can bind with hydrogen ion in the serum

   d. K+ can bind with bicarbonate in the serum

Answer: b. K+ is exchanged with hydrogen ion that goes into the cells to normalize the blood pH.

79. When lactate is increased in the serum, what acid base problem is noted?

   a. Metabolic alkalosis

   b. Respiratory acidosis

   c. Respiratory alkalosis

   d. Metabolic acidosis

Answer: d. Lactic acidosis is a type of metabolic acidosis caused by release of lactic acid from overused muscle cells.

80. In metabolic acidosis, what EKG finding is common?

   a. Flat T waves

   b. Tall peaked T waves

   c. Narrow QRS interval

d. No EKG findings are noted

Answer: b. Tall, peaked T waves are noted in metabolic acidosis because the serum potassium level is often increased.

81. A nursing intervention in metabolic acidosis if the pH is less than 7.2 includes what?

    a. Administer Calcium chloride by IV

    b. Administer NaOH by IV

    c. Administer NaHCO3 by IV

    d. Administer extra IV fluids to dilute out the pH

Answer: c. If the pH is below 7.2, Na-bicarbonate can be administered by IV to normalize the pH.

82. When administering NaHCO3 by IV, the line must be flushed before and after giving the sodium bicarbonate. Why is this so?

    a. It decreases the risk of metabolic alkalosis.

    b. Sodium bicarbonate precipitates with many medications

    c. Sodium bicarbonate can cause excessive heat when mixed with acidic medications.

    d. Sodium bicarbonate is irritating to the veins.

Answer: b. Sodium bicarbonate precipitates with many medications so the line must be flushed before and after giving sodium bicarbonate in an IV solution.

83. When sodium bicarbonate is given to reduce metabolic acidosis, what must be looked out for?

    a. Reduction in potassium levels

    b. Elevation in potassium levels

    c. Reduction in chloride levels

    d. Reduction in magnesium levels

Answer: a. When sodium bicarbonate is given, potassium will re-enter the cells, causing a reduction in potassium in the serum.

84. The first response to metabolic alkalosis is what?

    a. Hyperventilation to blow off CO_2.

    b. Increase in renal loss of HCO_3-.

    c. A decrease in renal loss of HCO_3-.

    d. Hypoventilation to hang onto CO_2.

Answer: d. The first response in metabolic alkalosis is a decrease in ventilations that hangs onto CO_2 in order to normalize the blood pH.

85. If a client has uncompensated metabolic alkalosis, what ABG findings are noted?

    a. pH elevated

    b. PCO_2 elevated

    c. HCO_3- is decreased

    d. pH is normal

Answer: a. If the patient has uncompensated metabolic alkalosis, the PCO2 is normal, the pH is elevated and the HCO3- level is increased.

86. A common cause of metabolic alkalosis is what?

    a. Elevated potassium level

    b. EKG changes

    c. Losses from GI suctioning

    d. Renal failure

Answer: c. If excess H+ is lost due to gastric suctioning, there will be metabolic alkalosis. Another cause of metabolic alkalosis is giving too much sodium bicarbonate in the IV.

87. A common treatment of metabolic alkalosis is what?

    a. Give HCl by IV.

    b. Give Diamox by IV to promote bicarbonate excretion by the kidneys

    c. Hyperventilate the patient.

    d. Give potassium chloride by IV.

Answer: b. Diamox can be given by IV in metabolic alkalosis in order to increase the bicarbonate excretion by the kidneys.

88. Which of the following clients is at the highest risk of hypernatremia?

    a. An elderly client with diaphoresis, high fever and pneumonia.

    b. An elderly CHF client on loop diuretics.

    c. A middle aged client with vomiting and diarrhea.

d. A sixty year old with SIADH.

Answer: a. A client who is sweating will lose more free water than sodium and is at a higher risk of hypernatremia. The others are likely to have low or normal sodium levels.

89. A client has treated diabetic ketoacidosis. The blood sugar is normal and the pH and serum osmolality are normal. Nevertheless, the client is experiencing leg weakness. What is a nursing priority?

a. Order physical therapy

b. Order a serum potassium level.

c. Have the patient rest throughout the day

d. Increase dairy products and calcium-containing leafy green vegetable intake.

Answer: a. When the diabetic ketoacidosis is resolved, the potassium can go back into the cells so that hypokalemia can result.

90. A client has an elevated potassium level and is scheduled to receive Kayexalate. After giving the Kayexelate, the nurse should monitor what?

a. The blood pressure

b. The urine output

c. The bowel movements

d. The EKG, looking for peaked T waves

Answer: c. The client with hyperkalemia needs to have bowel movements In order for the Kayexalate to be effective. The peaked T waves would be present before treatment and should resolve as long as the client has bowel movements.

91. A client with a serum K+ of 4.5 the day before has a repeat K+ of 7.0 the next day with no signs or symptoms of hyperkalemia. What is the next step?

    a. Administer Kayexalate.

    b. Redraw the blood.

    c. Increase the intake of bananas.

    d. Report the result to the physician.

Answer: b. If the client has no symptoms, the nurse must suspect that the blood draw had resulted in a hemolyzed specimen, which has elevated K+ due to red blood cell release of potassium.

92. A client is receiving IV magnesium to correct a magnesium deficit. What would the nurse look for as an indication to stop the infusion?

    a. A lack of patellar reflexes

    b. Premature ventricular contractions

    c. Diarrhea

    d. Blood pressure elevation

Answer: a. If the magnesium level gets too high, there will be a lack of patellar reflexes.

93. A client with chronic renal failure has lost ten pounds over the last three months. He has problems taking calcium supplements. The total calcium level is low. What is the next step?

    a. Check the reflexes.

    b. Report a very low calcium level to the physician.

    c. Prepare to give calcium gluconate.

    d. Check an albumin level.

Answer: d. If the client has lost weight, the albumin level might be low. This will result in a total lowering of the serum calcium level but likely a normal ionized serum calcium level.

94. A CHF client is complaining of nausea. He has just put out 2500 cc of urine after receiving Lasix. Which should be done before administering the digoxin? Check all that apply.

    a. Give Compazine before giving the digoxin.

    b. Increase fluid intake.

    c. Call the physician before giving the digoxin.

    d. Tell the physician about the urine output.

    e. Tell the physician about the nausea.

    f. Look for peaked T waves on EKG.

Answer: c. d. e. The patient may have hypokalemia from such a loss of urine. Call the physician to report the urine output and tell the physician about the symptoms. The digoxin should be held until the K+ has returned as low K+ can cause digoxin toxicity.

NCLEX Takeover

95. A client with multiple myeloma has a serum calcium level of 13 mg/dL. What should the nurse do?

    a. Encourage fluid intake and increase passive range of motion.

    b. Tell the client to increase nut and whole grain intake.

    c. Have a tracheostomy tray at the bedside

    d. Give calcium gluconate IM.

Answer: a. The calcium level is elevated. By increasing fluids and encouraging ROM, the calcium is allowed to go into the bone and through the kidneys. The tracheostomy tray should be encouraged in hypocalcemia and you shouldn't give calcium gluconate (especially not by IM means).

96. An elderly client does not recognize family members and has a sodium level of 113 mEq/L. What does the nurse tell the family members about the client's condition?

    a. The client is suffering from dementia.

    b. Older clients often get confused in the hospital.

    c. The sodium level is too low, resulting in these temporary symptoms.

    d. The sodium level is high and the client is dehydrated.

Answer: c. The sodium level is low so the client is confused and can be aggressive. When the sodium level normalizes, these symptoms will likely dissipate.

97. A client with a low sodium level is receiving 3 percent Normal Saline at 50 cc/hr over a 16 hour period of time. The client now feels short of breath and is fatigued. What nursing intervention should be done first?

   a. Turn down the IV.

   b. Check the sodium level.

   c. Check for fluid overload.

   d. Call the physician.

Answer: c. A client receiving IV fluid with sodium in it is at risk for fluid overload. Assess the patient for this condition before calling the physician or before even lowering the IV dose of sodium. A sodium level should be checked but not before assessing for fluid overload.

98. A client on dialysis complains of complication. What laxative should the client avoid taking?

   a. Dulcolax suppository

   b. High fiber supplements

   c. Docusate sodium

   d. Milk of Magnesia

Answer: d. A client on dialysis is at risk for magnesium overload. They should not take Milk of Magnesia, which contains magnesium.

99. The client is being given IV fluids with potassium. The urine output has been 120 cc per shift over the last two shifts. Before giving potassium again, what should the nurse do?

a. Encourage an increase in fluid intake.

b. Give the K+ as ordered.

c. Draw a K+ level and give the next dose if the K+ is low or normal.

d. Hold the next dose and call the physician.

Answer: d. The urine output is too low (below 30 cc per hour) so the patient is at risk for hyperkalemia. Call the physician for an order to get another K+ level before giving the next dose.

100. A client should be watched for low phosphorus levels in which situation?

a. A client on calcium and vitamin D who has osteoporosis.

b. An alcoholic client on TPN.

c. A client with chronic renal failure awaiting dialysis.

d. A client with low PTH due to thyroid surgery.

Answer: b. A client on TPN who is an alcoholic is at risk for low phosphorus levels. The others are at risk for high phosphorus levels.

101.　　　A client has pancreatitis and has been on potassium for 4 days for a low potassium level. Today the potassium level is still low. What lab value should the nurse check to see why the client is not responding to treatment?

a. Sodium

b. Phosphorus

c. Calcium

d. Magnesium

Answer: d. Low magnesium levels can interfere with potassium entering the cells. The magnesium level must be normalized before treatment for hypokalemia can work.

102.　　　A client has chronic renal failure. What should the nurse encourage the client to do?

a. Increase nuts and dairy products.

b. Take aluminum-based antacids after every meal

c. Reduce intake of meat, chocolate and whole grains

d. Avoid taking calcium supplements.

Answer: b. Aluminum-based antacids can help bind phosphorus and help it be eliminated through the GI tract so this is important in chronic renal failure.

103.　　　A client with COPD is short of breath on 2 l of O2 when doing little activity. The ABGs show pH of 7.36, PaCO2 62, HCO3 35, and O2 88 percent. What should the nurse do first?

a.　Call the physician to report the condition.

b.　Turn the O2 up to 4 lpm

c.　Have the client rest and take deep breaths

d.　Teach the client pursed lip breathing.

Answer: d. Pursed lip breathing is the best technique to improve shortness of breath in a compensated COPD patient with mild hypoxia.

104.　　　A postoperative client has been vomiting and experiences dizziness upon arising. The BP is 55/50 and the pulse is 140. What IV fluids should be given?

a.　D5W+0.45 NS at 50 cc per hour

b.　NS at open

c.　D5W at 125 cc per hour

d.　0.45 NS at open

Answer: b. The client probably need volume replacement which can best be given by using normal saline as fast as it can be run in until stable.

105.   A client has had an NG tube placed to low suction for the last 2 days. What should the nurse be on the lookout for?

a. Respiratory alkalosis

b. Respiratory acidosis

c. Metabolic alkalosis

d. Metabolic acidosis

Answer: c. The constant loss of H+ ions in NG suctioning can lead to metabolic alkalosis.

Conclusion

I hope you received a ton of value from this book. Remember, practice makes perfect so you will have to repeat these questions.

If you enjoyed this book, would you be kind enough to leave a review on Amazon? Your positive review can help others to see what kinds of helpful resources are out there!

Thank you and good luck on your medical endeavors!

- Chase Hassen

Recommended Books for Success

NCLEX: Respiratory System : 105 Nursing Practice Questions and Rationales to Easily Crush the NCLEX!

NCLEX: Endocrine System : 105 Nursing Practice Questions and Rationales to EASILY Crush the NCLEX!

NCLEX: Integumentary System: 105 Nursing Practice Questions and Rationales to EASILY Crush the NCLEX!

NCLEX: Emergency Nursing : 105 Practice Questions and Rationales to Easily Crush the NCLEX!

EKG Interpretation: 24 Hours or Less to Easily Pass the ECG Portion of the NCLEX!

Nursing Careers: Easily Choose What Nursing Career Will Make Your 12 Hour Shift a Blast!

Night Shift: 10 Survival Tips For Nurses to Get Through the Night!

Chase Hassen

Highly Recommended Books for Success

1. <u>NCLEX: Cardiovascular System : 105 Nursing Practice and Rationales to Easily Crush the NCLEX!</u>

2. <u>NCLEX: Emergency Nursing : 105 Practice Questions and Rationales to Easily Crush the NCLEX!</u>

3. <u>Lab Values: 137 Values You Know to Easily Pass The NCLEX!</u>

4. <u>EKG Interpretation: 24 Hours or Less to Easily Pass the ECG Portion of the NCLEX!</u>

5. <u>Fluid and Electrolytes: 24 Hours or Less to Absolutely Crush the NCLEX Exam!</u>

6. <u>Nursing Careers: Easily Choose What Nursing Career Will Make Your 12 Hour Shift a Blast!</u>

7. <u>Night Shift: 10 Survival Tips for Nurses to Get Through The Night!</u>

8. <u>NCLEX: Endocrine System : 105 Nursing Practice Questions and Rationales to EASILY Crush the NCLEX!</u>

And ***MUCH MUCH MORE***! Visit my amazon author page to see more at http://amzn.to/1HCtfSy

www.ingramcontent.com/pod-product-compliance
Lightning Source LLC
Chambersburg PA
CBHW051452170526
45166CB00001B/209